Cardiology for Student

Bryan Dowe

with all good wish

for

Dug

To

Greta, J and D.

Cardiology for Students

Max Zoob M.D., F.R.C.P.,

Consultant Cardiologist, Regional Cardiac Unit, Brook General Hospital,
London.

Foreword by J.F. Goodwin, M.D., F.R.C.P., F.A.C.C.
Professor of Clinical Cardiology, Consultant Physician, Royal
Postgraduate Medical School, London.

CHURCHILL LIVINGSTONE
Edinburgh London and New York 1979

CHURCHILL LIVINGSTONE

Medical Division of Longman Group Limited

Distributed in the United States of America by Longman Inc., 19 West 44th Street, New York, N.Y. 10036 and by associated companies, branches and representatives throughout the world.

ISBN 0 443 01530 9

Library of Congress Cataloging in Publication Data

Zoob, Max.
    Cardiology for students.

    Includes index.
    1.   Heart-Diseases.   2.   Cardiovascular system-Diseases.
I.   Title.   [DNLM: 1.   Heart diseases – Diagnosis.
WG141 Z87c]
RC681.Z66   616.1'2   76–54864

Printed in Singapore by
New Art Printing Co Pte Ltd

Foreword

The subject of cardiovascular disease has now become so vast and so sub-specialised that it is difficult to encompass it effectively within a textbook of medicine and difficult to know how much detail to include.

Dr Zoob's short textbook whets the appetite of the students and cardiovascular nurse and the same time provides a source for reference that is easily assimilable and effectively illustrated by simple drawings.

The style is straightforward and readable, the phraseology sometimes suggesting a nostalgia for the incisive style of the late Paul Wood, to whom Dr Zoob pays tribute in his preface. Dr Zoob has followed in general the format of Wood's classic textbook, beginning with structure and function and proceeding to symptoms, signs, investigations and then specific cardiovascular disorders.

The aim has been to concentrate on broad principles so that fine description of details of diagnosis and treatment are not to be expected.

In an era when the increasing complexity and sophistication of instrumentation threaten to overwhelm the clinician and sometimes obscure important basic clinical aspects the second chapter, which clearly describes symptoms and signs of cardiovascular disease, is particularly welcome and will be of great value to the student.

Dr Zoob is to be commended also for his handling of references. He has avoided the twin pitfalls of too extensive referencing on the one hand and total omission of all references on the other. Each chapter is followed by a short list for recommended reading.

The final section on actions and unwanted effects of drugs is a useful addition and could be expanded in future editions.

I have much pleasure in wishing Dr Zoob every success in this venture.

1978   J. F. Goodwin

Acknowledgements

It is a pleasure to acknowledge my indebtedness to the teachers who first interested me in cardiology and especially in the value and techniques of bedside observation. They include Sir George Pickering, the late Dr Paul Wood, Sir John McMichael, and Professor John Goodwin.

I am greatly indebted to my friend and colleague Dr E. Gaertner who has read the manuscript meticulously and helped me with much stimulating and constructive criticism and advice.

It is a pleasure to acknowledge the excellent work of Mr Frank Price who made the line drawings, and my secretaries Mrs P. Buxey and Mrs E. C. Mills.

I am grateful to Hoechst Pharmaceuticals for permission to adapt illustrations from their booklet on Echocardiography.

London, 1978   Max Zoob

Introduction

The last 30 years have seen remarkable changes both in the total incidence of heart disease and in the frequency of its various forms. The most spectacular alteration has been a nearly two-fold increase in coronary artery disease which has made cardiovascular disorders the commonest cause of death in the Western World. Another remarkable change, the significance of which is probably not yet fully apparent, has been the appearance of the primary cardiomyopathies as partially defined though at present fairly uncommon entities. At the same time the frequency of rheumatic and syphilitic heart disease has diminished strikingly. Consideration of incidence and frequency are particularly important in diagnosis, which is after all a question of probabilities. Common conditions are more likely to be encountered than rare ones and though the former may be reasonably diagnosed in the presence of some unusual or atypical features, the latter may not. Rarities should be thought of frequently but diagnosed rarely and then only on particularly secure grounds.

Incidence and frequency must of course be reflected in any textbook so that the amount of detail is related to the commonness of the disorder described. But this cannot be the sole criterion of proportions for several reasons. Thus rheumatic heart disease—though now much less common than ischeamic or hypertensive heart disease—merits a full presentation since this ensures a training in auscultation and haemodynamic concepts applicable to the whole of cardiology. The same is true to a lesser extent of congenital heart disease which is comparatively rare. Again, a knowledge of the cardiomyopathies should draw attention to the considerable numbers of patients with florid heart disease whose aetiology is totally unknown. This should lead to a preoccupation with aetiological diagnosis and help to eradicate the prevalent habit of thinking of 'congestive heart failure' as a complete diagnosis. It should also discourage the habit of making a facile diagnosis of a common condition in a patient lacking some of its usual signs or presenting unusual ones—rarities should be considered frequently though diagnosed rarely.

These were some of the considerations which determined the proportions of this book. Short sections usually imply uncommon disorders and when a larger section has been devoted to them their relative frequency has been noted.

Contents

Acknowledgements

Introduction

1 The Structure and Properties of Heart Muscle
  and Heart Failure 1

2 Symptoms and Signs 15

3 Haemodynamics 46

4 Radiology 54

5 Echocardiography 63

6 Electrocardiography 70

7 The Heart Rate and Rhythm and the Dysrhythmias 99

8 Disorders of Conduction 120

9 High Blood Pressure 129

10 Phaeochromocytoma 142

11 Ischaemic Heart Disease 145

12 Congenital Heart Disease 177

13 Rheumatic Fever 201

14 Diseases of the Heart Valves 209

15 Hyperkinetic Circulatory States 236

16 Bacterial Endocarditis 239

17 Pericarditis 245

18 Pericardial Constriction 250

19 Myxoma of the Atria 253

20 Pulmonary Embolism 255

21 Pulmonary Hypertension 264

22 Chronic Cor Pulmonale 269

23 Dissecting Aneurysm of the Aorta 274

24 The Cardiomyopathies 278

25 Resuscitation 284

26 Anxiety State with Cardiovascular Symptoms 287

27 Action of Drugs 290

1. The Structure and Properties of Heart Muscle and Heart Failure

Throughout biology, structure can be seen to be intimately related to function and study of the one enhances understanding of the other.

In recent years electron microscopy of heart muscle cells (fibres) has revealed the structural basis for some of the fundamental properties of heart muscle. Each muscle cell is composed of longitudinal fibrils which are divided by dark transverse bands (Z lines) into the individual basic units of contraction, the sarcomeres, whose structure is shown in Fig. 1.1. Thin (50 Å diam.) actin filaments arise from the Z lines,

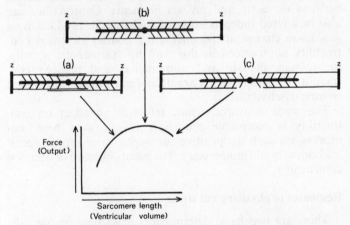

Fig. 1.1 The relationship between structure and function of the sarcomere (see text). (a) The sarcomere is insufficiently stretched so that the overlapping parts of the actin fibrils cannot be engaged by the bridges of the myosin filaments. The force and output developed is submaximal and the muscle is operating on the ascending limb of Starling's curve shown below. (b) At the peak of the curve stretching is optimal and all the bridges are engaged. (c) The sarcomere is overstretched and some of the bridges are disengaged. Developed force is sub-optimal corresponding to the falling limb of the curve.

interdigitate with the thicker (100 Å diam.) centrally placed myosin filaments and are connected to them by bridges. During contraction the Z lines approximate and although the cells shorten the actin and myosin filaments do not. They must therefore slide over one another, impelled it is thought by forces generated at the points of contact of the bridges. The maximum force of contraction occurs when all the bridges are operative (Fig. 1.1(b)). If the muscle is stretched too little, the ends of the actin filaments overlap and cannot be engaged, while if it is overstretched some bridges are disengaged (Fig. 1.1(a) & (c)). This is the ultra-structural basis for the physiological observation embodied in Starling's Law, that the force of contraction increases with fibre length until the latter is optimal, and then diminishes (Braunwald 1971). The term myocardial contractility refers to the force and velocity of contraction of the myocardium; its alteration by a change in preliminary stretching (pre-load), just described, depends on a *quantitative* change in the number of interacting points between the actin and myosin filaments. Contractility can also be altered independently of a change in pre-load by a *qualitative* change at the interacting points; increased contractility is produced in this way by sympathetic activity, tachycardia, digoxin and isoprenaline, and reduced contractility by beta-blocking agents and most of the drugs used to treat dysrhythmias.

The word inotropic, which refers to an effect on contractility is acceptable though it is not used here, but expressions such as 'positive (or negative) inotropic agent' are both ugly and unnecessary. The agents increase or decrease contractility.

Responses to physiological stress

There are two basic determinants of cardiac output—the heart rate and the stroke volume. The heart rate is governed by vagal activity which tends to slow it and by sympathetic activity mediated by the catecholamines adrenaline and noradrenaline. These tend to increase the rate and also increase the force and velocity of contractions. Probably sympathetic and para-sympathetic effects work in harmony to produce changes in cardiac output; thus increased vagal activity and diminution of catechol amine production may reduce the heart rate and cardiac output during sleep. An increased cardiac output which occurs normally after food, on emotion, stooping, or during exercise is probably mediated mainly by the sympathetic nervous system through an increased production of catecholamines. The contrasting actions of adrenaline, noradrenaline, isoprenaline and their antagonists are shown in Table 1.1. It will be seen that

Table 1.1 The effects of catecholamines and drugs blocking α and β sympathetic receptors with the resultant effects on the circulation.

| Compound | Action on Sympathetic Receptors | | | Result |
	Heart (β)	Peripheral Vessels constriction (α)	dilatation (β)	
Noradrenaline	+	+ +	−	B.P. ↑ Periph: Flow ↓ Cardiac Output Unchanged Systolic Pressure ↑ Diastolic Pressure ↓
Adrenaline	+ +	+	+ +	Muscle Flow ↑ Skin Flow ↓ Cardiac Output ↑ Systolic Pressure ↑ Diastolic Pressure ↓
Isoprenaline	+ + +	−	+ + +	Peripheral Flow ↑ Cardiac Output ↓
Propranolol	Blocks			Heart Slowed ↑ Cardiac Output ↓
Phentolamine	−	Blocks	−	Vasodilatation B.P. ↓ Cardiac Output ↓

noradrenaline causes generalized vasoconstriction affecting the arteries of muscle, heart and skin, with a total increase in vascular resistance and pressure and reflex slowing of the heart. By contrast, adrenaline produces effects ideally suited to the increased cardiac output required during exercise and other physiological activities. It increases the heart rate, dilates the arteries of the heart and muscles where extra blood flow is required and it constricts the skin vessels where increased flow is not needed. As a result the total vascular resistance falls, the systolic blood pressure rises and the diastolic pressure falls. The cardiac output increases so that the venous return increases, increasing the filling pressure of the right heart thus increasing the force of contraction of the right ventricle, according. to Starling's law. The left atrium and ventricle follow suit in due course with a resultant further increase in cardiac output. An increased contractility results from the increased sympathetic activity. It has been observed that dynamic exercise involving movement of the body such as walking and running produces relatively slight increases in cardiac work and blood pressure while static work such as maintaining weight against gravity or tasks involving straining or gripping causes a great increase in blood pressure and a correspondingly large increase in cardiac work. This is highly relevant to the type of exercise and work which should be allowed to patients suffering or convalescent from heart disease. They can usually be permitted to engage in dynamic forms of work and exercise but it may be necessary to advise against or restrict static exercises or work involving heavy static strain.

These normal mechanisms of increasing cardiac output can be altered by drugs, especially those which block the beta adrenergic receptors. Propranolol is the best established of ˙ese; it reduces the heart rate and decreases the force of contraction. Isoprenaline is a powerful beta receptor stimulant increasing the heart rate and force of contraction and dilating skeletal blood vessels and bronchi. Phenoxy-benzamine (phentolamine) blocks the alpha-receptors leading to vasolilatation in the skin and it also stimulates production of catechol amines so that there is increased cardiac output with fall of blood pressure and dilatation of the bronchi. The action of these drugs is summarised in Table 1.1.

Response to pathological stresses

There are two main categories of pathological stress:
1. Increased volume work
2. Increased pressure work

Increased volume work is demanded of the heart if any of its valves leak. Then, if a normal quantity of blood is to be delivered to the body, the heart must pump an additional amount corresponding to that which leaks back through the faulty valve. Increased volume work is also demanded of the heart if there is an abnormal congenital communication between the left and right sides of the heart allowing a shunt or short-circuit in the circulation. Then too, if a normal volume is to be delivered to the body an additional quantity must be pumped by the heart corresponding to the quantity taking the shortened route. This is explained in detail in the chapter on haemodynamics.

Whatever the cause the heart responds to the increased volume load by increased force of contraction, according to Starling's law. The dilatation becomes permanent and is followed by hypertrophy. The filling pressure rises proportionately. The rapid filling of a dilated ventricle which is the essential feature of the condition gives characteristic clinical findings. The ventricle can be felt to have a large amplitude pulsation (a hyperkinetic ventricle). The rapid filling produces an audible 3rd sound in the first third of diastole (p. 35).

The increased diastolic pressure is communicated to the atrium and to the venous and capillary territories up-stream with consequences described under left and right heart failure in subsequent pages. Although dilatation of the ventricle produces increased force of contraction it is not without disadvantages. Laplace showed that the greater the cavity size the greater is the wall tension needed to produce a given intraventricular pressure. The reduced efficiency of the dilated ventricle is shown by the increased oxygen requirement needed for a given amount of heart work and a reduced rate of rise of intraventricular pressure.

The heart performs increased pressure work when it is forced to eject against increased resistance as in systemic or pulmonary hypertension or when there is obstruction at the aortic or pulmonary valves. The heart responds by hypertrophy—its individual fibres thickening and lengthening. Although the ratio between capillaries and fibres appears to remain one to one, some difficulty of diffusion of oxygen from the capillary to the centre of the cell may occur as the cell becomes very thick with some consequent impairment of function. Hypertrophied muscle is uncompliant and tends to resist stretching. A powerful atrial contraction is needed to ensure adequate filling. This may produce an audible presystolic sound which together with a powerful but small amplitude thrust are the characteristic clinical findings of a ventricle performing excessive pressure work (a hyperdynamic ventricle). The pressure, at first raised only during atrial contraction in pre-systole, later becomes elevated throughout diastole and this elevated pressure is transmitted from the ventricle to atrium and venous and capillary territories with consequences described below.

Heart failure

It is remarkable but true that there is no satisfactory definition of heart failure. It has been stated to mean an inability of the heart to pump sufficient blood to meet the normal requirements of the body. The latter however cannot be defined, and surely if the normal requirements are not met the patient must die. Failure cannot be defined simply in terms of cardiac output or cardiac index (output per square metre of body surface area). These measurements may fall within the wide normal range although the patient shows the clinical features generally accepted as those of heart failure. A definition which is clinically applicable was that proposed by Sharpey Shafer who emphasised that the failing heart is unable to adjust its output to an altered inflow. This can be demonstrated at the bedside by asking the patient to perform the Valsalva manoeuvre in which he expires forcibly against a closed glottis with the nostrils held closed. This manoeuvre abruptly reduces the venous return to the heart which normally responds with a diminution of cardiac output, reduction of the stroke volume and consequent fall in pulse pressure. The reduction of stroke volume can be felt at the brachial or radial pulse and the reduction in pulse pressure can be measured with a sphygmomanometer. On release of the forced expiratory effort there is a sudden increase of stroke volume, pulse pressure and heart rate. If there is heart failure these parameters are unchanged by the manoeuvre which simply increases the systolic and diastolic arterial pressure owing to the rise in intra-thoracic pressure.

In addition however to this useful and attractive definition the more widely understood and accepted sense of the term 'congestive heart failure' and 'left' and 'right heart failure' must be described. The terms imply the presence of raised pulmonary or systemic venous pressure together with the presence of pulmonary or systemic oedema consequent on water and salt retention. Formerly it was thought that the mechanism was quite simple. The pressure was presumed to rise behind the 'failing ventricle' so that the venous and capillary pressures rose exceeding the osmotic pressures and therefore caused transudation in the extra-cellular compartment and hence oedema. Subsequently however it was found that in many cases water and salt retention preceded the rise of venous pressure which followed secondarily. Sometimes the two events occurred almost simultaneously. The mechanism of the salt and water retention has still not been fully elucidated. The reduction in the glomerular filtration fraction seems to be only a minor factor and increased tubular reabsorption of sodium through the action of aldosterone can be detected only in a proportion of severe cases. However these mechanisms may be present transiently in mild cases but disappear before they are detected. The distribution of the oedema probably depends on the site of elevation of the venous pressures. If there has been a pressure or volume load on the left ventricle as in hypertension or mitral reflux, the left atrial and pulmonary venous pressures are raised and pulmonary oedema usually occurs when the pulmonary venous pressure exceeds the normal osmotic pressure of 25 to 30 mmHg. Persistently raised pulmonary capillary pressure may cause a slow transudation of fluid into the alveolar walls which become fibrosed so that higher pressures may be tolerated before pulmonary oedema occurs. When it does however, the result is the same, serous fluid seeps into the alveolar walls and thence into the alveoli themselves to be coughed up by the patient as pink frothy sputum. The clinical picture is described below.

If the pressure or volume load has been on the right ventricle as in pulmonary hypertension or atrial septal defect the systemic venous pressure is raised as can be appreciated by inspection of the jugular veins, and the liver is enlarged. Oedema develops in the dependant parts where the hydrostatic pressure exceeds the colloid osmotic pressure; ascites and pleural effusions may develop by a similar mechanism.

Pulmonary oedema is commonly referred to as 'left ventricular failure' and oedema with raised venous pressure, liver enlargement and perhaps pleural effusions, is often referred to as 'right ventricular failure'. These terms however are unfortunate. It has previously been noted that the cardiac output is not always below normal when these features are present; indeed in many cases the *work* of the heart is actually increased. For example, in arterial hypertension the blood pressure often rises during an attack of pulmonary oedema and if the output is normal the heart is performing greatly increased work. Oedema results from the very high pulmonary venous pressure. Similarly on the right side severe pulmonary hypertension and tricuspid reflux greatly increase the work of the heart which is actually contracting extremely forcefully at a time when oedema develops and right heart *failure* is said to be present. It would therefore seem much better simply to speak of pulmonary or systenic oedema and to state their cause.

The direct impairment of myocardial function

Myocardial function may be directly impaired in two ways, the myocardium may be affected by disease or its effective working may be hampered by disease of the pericardium or rarely the endocardium.

a. *Myocardial disease*. The most common is ischaemic disease resulting from coronary artery atheroma. Infarction or diffuse fibrosis reduces the contractile power of the left ventricle. Other disorders reducing the contractility of the muscles include myxoedema, amyloid disease, haemochromatosis and other metabolic cardiomyopathies and hypertrophic cardiomyopathies of unknown cause. Cardiomyopathies are also associated with hereditary neurological myopathies. Cardiac and vascular responses to the impairment of myocardial function produced by these disorders is similar to those produced by increased pathological loads already described. There is increased diastolic volume with increased filling pressure in order to maintain cardiac output. This is accompanied by an audible third heart sound or gallop rhythm. The heart is clinically and radiologically enlarged and hypertrophy may follow. Water and salt retention ensues and there may be pulmonary or dependent oedema with the clinical features described below.

b. *Pericardial constriction or effusion*. This may severely impair filling of the heart. The pulmonary venous pressure and the systemic venous pressure rise to a great height but the heart, encased by dense fibrous tissue or surrounded by incompressible fluid within the pericardial sac, cannot enlarge to accommodate entering blood and its output is therefore limited and fixed. Sodium and water retention follow with consequent oedema and often ascites and pleural effusions. The high venous pressure results in gross liver enlargement. The clinical picture closely resembles that due to 'right heart failure' but in pericardial constriction the heart is small.

Pulmonary oedema

Definition. Transudation of fluid from capillaries into the alveolar walls and alveolar spaces of the lungs.

Mechanism and causes. Transudation may occur when the hydrostatic pressure exceeds the colloid osmotic pressure of about 25 mmHg. The normal mean left atrial pressure is below 12 mmHg. It is elevated if the left atrium has difficulty in emptying. This is the case if the left ventricle is uncompliant due to hypertrophy. The causes of hypertrophy include hypertension and aortic valve disease. The left ventricular end-diastolic pressure may be raised through myocardial disease, including myocardial infarction and cardiomyopathy and this would of course be communicated to the left atrium, pulmonary veins and capillaries. The left atrial pressure would also be elevated by mitral reflux and mitral stenosis and rarely too by a ball thrombus or myxoma obstructing the mitral valve. The exact level of pressure at which pulmonary oedema occurs is variable. If the left atrial pressure and pulmonary capillary pressure are persistently elevated to the colloid osmotic pressure of 25 mmHg, a slow transudation of fluid into the alveolar wall may occur, leading to thickening and fibrosis which tends to prevent further exudation until higher pressures are reached. By contrast if there is a sudden increase of pressure above the critical value of 25 mmHg oedema occurs abruptly. Any sudden elevation of pressure such as occurs on exercise, emotion, sexual intercourse or increase in circulating blood volume as in pregnancy, may be the precipitating factor which leads to pulmonary oedema. Tachycardia, whether of sinus origin or due to an ectopic rhythm, is another precipitating factor because it shortens diastole and increases the venous pressure.

Clinical features. Sometimes but by no means invariably there is a history of progressive effort dyspnoea. The attack commonly occurs during the night, the patient being awakened by breathlessness or cough which rapidly worsens; he finds some relief by standing upright and often goes to an open window. Frequently he coughs up pink, frothy sputum and respiration may be noisy with wheeze. The patient is clearly distressed and respiration is laboured with the accessory muscles of respiration in use. The jugular venous pressure is hard to assess and the peripheral pulse is rapid and small in volume. Widespread crepitations over the lungs are characteristic but sometimes rhonchi are more conspicuous as in bronchial asthma. Depending on the cause there may be evidence of left ventricular hypertrophy with gallop rhythm or signs of mitral valve disease, but auscultatory observations are difficult to make in the presence of the respiratory distress.

The cardiogram. The cardiogram may show evidence of the underlying cause, namely a dysrhythmia, left ventricular hypertrophy or cardiac infarction. Mitral disease may be suspected if there are broad P waves due to left atrial enlargement, or if there is right ventricular hypertrophy due to pulmonary hypertension.

Radiology. In addition to the characteristic appearances of pulmonary oedema (p. 55). There may be signs pointing to the underlying disease, namely left ventricular enlargement or enlargement of the pulmonary artery and left atrium.

Diagnosis. It is important and often difficult to differentiate bronchial asthma. There is usually a history of less severe attacks extending over a period of years. The attack is marked by *expiratory* difficulty and the motionless attitude of the patient. The chest is held in an inspiratory position and he clutches for some support while visibly attempting to *expel* air from his chest with audible wheeze. Cardiac dullness to percusssion is absent and signs of heart disease are lacking. The blood pressure is not raised but there may be striking inspiratory diminution of pulse volume (misnamed pulsus paradoxus, see p. 246). The cardiogram would show only sinus tachycardia and perhaps some right axis deviation with possibly tall pointed P waves. An X-ray of the chest may show emphysema but usually a normal sized heart. Differentiation of the two conditions is extremely important because Morphine which is extremely valuable in cardiac cases is very dangerous in bronchial asthma.

Treatment. The treatment is an emergency and usually should not wait upon the cardiogram or radiology, provided that differentiation from bronchial asthma is reasonably certain. Morphine 10 to 20 mg should be given intramuscularly or intravenously provided there is no respiratory failure. High concentrations of oxygen should be given, if possible under slightly positive pressure, and tourniquets can be applied to three limbs to reduce the venous return to the heart. The tourniquets should be released every fifteen minutes and moved in a 'clock-wise' direction to the adjacent limb.

Aminophylline 0.25 g intravenously is often very effective and later Frusemide 20 to 80 mg intravenously can be very helpful. If the blood pressure is high it can be lowered quickly with intravenous Diazoxide 300 mg in an intravenous infusion.

'Congestive heart failure'

This is a common mode of termination of many forms of heart disease. There is elevation of the venous pressure in both pulmonary and systemic circuits with salt and water retention and oedema of the lungs and body. The former leads to breathlessness and a high pressure in the venous territories of the pleural cavities, peritoneum and liver causes pleural effusions, hepatic enlargement and ascites as well as dependent oedema. In the early stages there may be orthopnoea and paroxysmal nocturnal dyspnoea, if there is a left-sided lesion causing a high left atrial pressure. Nocturnal dyspnoea may be explained as follows. The left atrium is centrally placed with regard to its venous territory and posture therefore makes little difference to its filling pressure. By contrast the right atrium is asymmetrical with regard to its venous territory, as two thirds of the body lie caudal and only one third cephalad to it; on recumbency there is therefore a great increase in venous return from the lower two thirds of the body and a correspondingly increased output to the lungs. The left ventricle slowly responds by increasing its output as well but only at the expense of a further increase in pulmonary venous and capillary pressures, which makes the lungs turgid and causes acute breathlessness. The patient's immediate reaction is to adopt the upright position which reduces the output of the right heart and facilitates respiration. Later in the course of the disease when the right heart is less responsive to changes in inflow, these reactions do not occur and orthopnoea is less striking.

The clinical picture of congestive failure is easily recognized. The patient is often orthopneic and breathless at rest. The jugular venous pressure is raised and the pulse is small, rapid and often irregular due to atrial fibrillation. The heart is enlarged usually with bi-ventricular hypertrophy and there is gallop rhythm, or the murmurs of rheumatic heart disease. The liver is enlarged and there is dependent oedema. There may also be pleural effusions and ascites. In constrictive pericarditis many of these features are present but the heart is small and usually impalpable. The amplitude of the jugular pulse is very small though the 'y' dip may be pronounced. There may be a paradoxical fall in the jugular pressure with expiration and the peripheral arterial pulse may show an exaggeration of the normal diminution of pulse pressure with inspiration (erroneously called 'pulsus paradoxus'). (p.246).

Treatment. Attention is directed to the following points:

1. Improvement or treatment of the underlying disease, such as thyrotoxicosis, anaemia or critical mitral valve disease.

2. Control of Dysrhythmias

3. Reduction of the work of the heart by reducing physical activity. Rest in a large comfortable armchair reduces the cardiac output because of the upright position and movement of the legs is encouraged to guard against venous thrombosis.

4. Increase of myocardial contractility by the use of Digoxin.

5. Increased sodium and water excretion by diuretics.

Digoxin (p.295). Any of the regimes described may be used. The intravenous route is rarely indicated. The oral route is effective within one to three hours and has a peak affect in six to twelve hours. This is adequate in most cases. By the intravenous route, Digoxin is effective within fifteen minutes and has a peak effect in about two hours. Recently it has been found that the heavy loading dose described in the dose regimes is not always essential and that a balance between absorption and excretion is achieved within about seven days on 0.25 mg thrice daily. Special dose regimes are used for children and the elderly or if Digoxin has already been given. Careful watch is kept for toxic affects described on page 296. The effectiveness of Digoxin treatment can be judged by the fall in heart rate, which is conspicuous in atrial fibrillation but also occurs in sinus rhythm due to the improvement in cardiac efficiency. A striking diuresis is often produced.

Diuretics. In the acute phase Frusemide is the diuretic of choice in a dosage of 40 to 80 mg by mouth. If the condition is considered urgent, 20 to 80 mg can be given intra-muscularly or intravenously and potassium supplements should be given at this time. In refractory cases as much as 180 mg can be given in a single dose, and in massive unresponsive oedema it is sometimes necessary to add Aldactone to antagonise Aldosterone and at the same time conserve potassium. In such cases the oedema may have to be drained directly by allowing the legs to hang dependent for several hours and then puncturing them with Southey's tubes and allowing the fluid to drain into a bowl. As the patient improves, treatment with the milder thiazide diuretics or Chlorthalidone can be substituted for Frusemide, and increased physical activity can be allowed. Sometimes residual collections of fluid in the pleural cavity or ascites may have to be removed by direct drainage. With the use of potent diuretics severe restriction of salt intake may cause serious depletion of salt and chloride and is not advised. In resistant oedema, however salt should not be added to meals. Throughout the period of active treatment of heart failure the serum electrolytes should be estimated frequently, as they may undergo rapid changes during the period of diuresis, and this may in turn cause intoxication by Digoxin. At the end of the acute phase, the physician must ask himself what is the minimum therapy that is really required. Digoxin will usually be indicated but the amount of diuretics needed is very variable. As a general rule Frusemide is not a drug for maintainance therapy and a thiazide diuretic once or twice a week without Potassium supplement may be enough. Careful experiment to determine the minimum amount of maintainance therapy will save much needless expense and inconvenience.

FURTHER READING

Braunwald, E. (1971) Structure and function of the normal myocardium *British Heart Journal*, **33** (Supp), 3.

Brutsaert, D.L. & Sonnenblick, E.H. (1973) Cardiac muscle mechanics in the evaluation of myocardial contractility and pump function. *Progress in Cardiovascular Disease*, **16**, 337.

2. Symptoms and Signs

While a narrative history is being obtained from the patient, special attention is directed to the following seven cardinal symptoms of cardiovascular disease:

Dyspnoea
Chest pain
Palpitations
Haemoptysis
Syncope
Claudication
Oedema

An attempt should be made to grade the severity of all symptoms and to determine whether they are improving or worsening.

Dyspnoea

This may be defined as an unpleasant awareness of the need to breathe. It may be graded as follows:

Grade 1	Minimal	— Undue breathlessness on running
Grade 2A	Slight	— Undue breathlessness on hills, stairs, or heavy housework such as polishing
Grade 2B	Moderate	— Undue breathlessness on walking a level mile or light housework
Grade 3	Considerable	— Breathlessness on walking 50 yds or less.
Grade 4	Gross	— Breathlessness at rest.

Paroxysmal nocturnal dysponoea is a special variety of breathlessness which characteristically awakes the patient from sleep and causes him to pace restlessly about the room or stand at an open window in a vain effort to obtain relief.

It is often accompanied by an irritative cough and sometimes by the expectoration of frothy or blood-stained sputum. It may be caused by mitral stenosis or by conditions elevating the left ventricular diastolic pressure such as Hypertension or aortic valve disease. Differentiation from bronchial asthma is difficult and the features of the two conditions may be identical. The most constant difference is the restlessness of the cardiac patient contrasting with the motionless posture of the asthmatic leaning forward, visibly intent on *expelling* the air from his chest. Wheeziness and rhonchi may be found in both conditions, although they are commoner in bronchial asthma.

Chest pain

This is one of the commonest problems in medical practice and the cause and nature of it can frequently be elucidated by careful interrogation of the patient. Particular attention must be paid to four points:
1. Site and radiation
2. Quality
3. Relation to increased heart work
4. Duration

The characteristics of ischaemic cardiac pain are described later (p. 151), but it may be noted that many of them can be produced by disease of other intrathoracic structures. One feature alone infallibly indicates that the pain is due to cardiac ischaemia, namely a constant relationship between heart work and pain. Increased cardiac work caused by exercise, emotion, food, or vasoconstriction due to cold, produces pain and removal of these factors relieves it. The response to drugs such as Trinitrate is hard to evaluate and often misleading.

Left infra-mammary pain due to an anxiety state may occur in two forms. It may be a momentary, sharp, stabbing, knife-like pain occurring on effort, or a dull heavy aching pain occurring independently of exercise or other factors which increase cardiac work.

Palpitations

These imply a consciousness of the heart action as a

thumping or fluttering sensation in the chest. It should be determined whether the symptom occurs on effort or at rest, and whether it begins and ends abruptly or gradually. If the patient is asked to imitate the sensation by tapping on the chest, the approximate rate, regularity and duration can often be assessed. The frequency of the attacks and the accompaniment of breathlessness or pain should also be ascertained.

Haemoptysis

The following varieties may be encountered. A sudden profuse haemoptysis in an apparently healthy individual occurs in the early stages of mitral stenosis whereas staining of the sputum following an attack of bronchitis occurs later in that disease. Dark red blood brought up a day or so after the onset of pleural pain suggests pulmonary infarction, and pink, frothy sputum is pathognomonic of pulmonary oedema.

Syncope

Syncope on effort may result from sudden failure of the ventricle proximal to a narrowed valve as in pulmonary or aortic stenosis. Syncope occurring at rest as well as on exercise may be due to dysrhythmia or to heart block. In the latter case convulsions may accompany the attack but loss of consciousness is usually only a matter of a minute or less and recovery is rapid and complete.

On the other hand, a simple vaso-vagal faint always occurs when the patient is standing. It may be caused by violent emotion or fatigue, or prolonged immobility, as for example, in soldiers on parade. Other cardiac causes of syncope, which will be described in the following pages, include cyanotic congenital heart disease, ball thrombus of the left atrium with mitral stenosis, and intracardiac myxoma. It will be apparent that in only two of the conditions mentioned, is the diagnosis likely to depend solely upon the history, namely dysrhythmia and transient heart block. In the former, a history of palpitations preceding the attack or occurring apart from it is helpful, but in the latter the main difficulty is differentiation from epilepsy. In heart block, however, the duration of unconsciousness is shorter than in epilepsy, complete recovery is more rapid, and the cardiogram is likely to show a residual abnormality although the electro-encephalogram will not do so.

Claudication

The patient should be asked whether a cramp-like pain occurs in the legs on walking. If so can he 'walk it off' or is he forced to stand still? Does a similar pain occur in bed at night? The presence of these symptoms indicates peripheral arterial disease which is commonly accompanied by coronary artery disease and may modify the clinical picture and treatment of the latter.

Oedema

This is more correctly described as a physical sign, but the patient's observation of it may help to date its onset. The milder grades of it are not noticed by the patient but if it is more severe it may be observed in the evenings. Only if it is gross will it be apparent on rising in the mornings as well as during the day. It is usually but not invariably symmetrical in distribution.

Personal habits

In addition to a detailed family history and past medical history, the patient's personal habits and home background should be enquired into fully. Knowledge of his use of tobacco and alcohol, both past and present, his hours of work and sleep, and family responsibilities, will together provide a background against which symptoms can be evaluated. The need for modification of the daily routine may then become apparent, and the urgency of the need to relieve him of physical handicaps can be assessed.

The interpretation of the history

In evaluating the history, three important rules must always be observed.

1. *The patient's story must be believed.*

Malingering is very rare in this country in normal circumstances and the patient almost always tells the truth as it appears to him. It is astonishing how frequently physicians disbelieve or disregard the history simply because it points to a diagnosis which is considered improbable on other grounds.

2. *If the history is characteristic of organic disease it must be accepted as such, even though unsupported by instrumental and physical findings.*

These three methods of diagnosis must be given equal weight because the history alone, or the cardiogram alone, or rarely physical examination alone, may be sufficient for a correct diagnosis. However, the findings of the three procedures usually complement one another and any discrepancy between them should be critically examined. This may lead to the discovery either of errors of observation or interpretation, or the presence of unsuspected complications.

3. *Symptoms of psychogenic origin differ sharply from those of organic disease.*

They are no less real to the patient and must be accounted for.

Neglect of these elementary rules is all too common and leads to dangerous mistakes.

Physical signs. The whole body and urine must be examined but special attention is given to the following points.

General appearance

Diagnosis should begin as the patient enters the room or the physician approaches the bed. As the clinical history unfolds, possible diagnoses should suggest themselves, as much from what the patient says as from his general appearance. An agitated manner and over-emphatic description of symptoms suggest an anxiety state while a plain unvarnished tale suggests organic disease. Protuberance of the eyes may indicate thyrotoxicosis or cor pulmonale. Puffiness beneath the eyes should cause suspicion of myxoedema. Anaemia, polycythaemia, cyanosis and clubbing may be recognisable at a glance. Breathlessness interfering with speech will probably be found to have an organic cause, but its occurrence only in the pauses suggests neurotic hyperventilation.

Exaggerated arterial pulsation over the carotid arteries may be due to high blood pressure or excitement, but also occurs in conditions which cause a 'leak' from the aorta such as aortic valve reflux and patent ductus arteriosus. If the arterial pulsation is confined to the suprasternal notch it suggests a high atheromatous aorta in adults, while in children and young adults it is pathognomonic of coarctation of the aorta. Venous pulsation evident in the sitting position suggests heart failure.

These preliminary observations may point to the need for amplification of certain aspects of the history or orient subsequent examination towards the most rewarding lines of approach.

The hands

Coolness of the hands may result from local vaso-constriction due to cold or from a general vaso-constriction which may be due to a low cardiac output. Warmth of the hands suggests a high cardiac output. Finger clubbing, if due to heart disease, suggests a congenital defect if the patient is cyanosed and bacterial endocarditis if he is not.

The radial or brachial pulse

It is time that practitioners and nurses gave up the practice of counting the pulse. It is the heart rate which is important and this can only be reliably determined by auscultation. The most significant features to observe when feeling the pulse are the amplitude and wave form.

A large amplitude suggests a high cardiac output or an aortic leak. It denies the presence of a serious obstructive lesion or implies that if there is one there must be an associated complication (e.g. mitral stenosis with thyrotoxicosis). A small pulse amplitude is found when the cardiac output is low as in heart failure. It is also found if the circulation is obstructed by narrowing of the pulmonary arterioles or narrowing of one or more of the heart valves. A small pulse also occurs in mitral or tricuspid reflux and in conditions causing a reduced circulating blood volume.

The wave form of the pulse can be assessed by considering the rate of rise and fall of each pulse beat. A quick-rising or 'water-hammer' pulse occurs in the same conditions which cause a large pulse-amplitude. A slow-rising or 'anacrotic' pulse is characteristic of aortic stenosis. A quick rising pulse reaches its peak in about 0.1 sec; a normal pulse in 0.16 sec and a slow-rising pulse in 0.2 to 0.25 sec (Fig. 2.1). An impression of these differences, which are readily detectable with practice, can be gained by comparing the sound of a camera shutter set in turn to each of these three speeds.

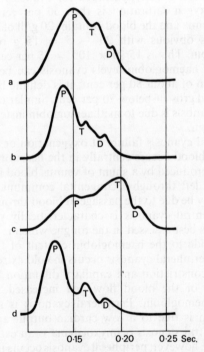

Fig. 2.1 *Diagram of a graphic record of the normal arterial pulse* (a) Each pulse shows three waves, the percussion wave (P), the tidal wave (T) and the dicrotic wave (D) caused by recoil from the closed aortic valve. (b) The quick-rising, large volume pulse is characteristic of aortic reflux and patent ductus arteriosus. It reaches its peak in about 0.1 seconds. (c) The slow-rising small volume pulse is characteristic of aortic stenosis. It takes more than 0.18 sec to peak and has a pronounced 'shoulder' on the upstroke. (d) The pulse in obstructive cardiomyopathy (p. 280) rises sharply, but the volume is small because muscular hypertrophy obstructs the out-flow from the left ventricle causing the pulse to collapse in late systole.

Cyanosis

A bluish discolouration of the skin or mucosae can be suspected if the amount of reduced haemoglobin in the capillaries is about 3 g/dl and is obvious if it is 5 g/dl. There is, however, only an indirect relationship between the appearances of cyanosis and oxygen saturation. If there is anaemia and the blood contains only 10 g/dl of haemoglobin, half of it must be unoxygenated for cyanosis to be definite and the oxygen saturation is then 50 per cent. If there is polycythaemia and the blood contains 20 g/dl of haemoglobin, cyanosis is obvious with $20 - 5 = 15$ g of oxygenated haemoglobin. This is $15/20 \times 100 = 75$ per cent saturation. At normal haemoglobin levels cyanosis can be suspected at a saturation of about 80 per cent; it is definite between 70–80 per cent and gross if below 70 per cent. Similar considerations apply if cyanosis is due to methaemoglobin instead of reduced haemoglobin.

In central cyanosis failure of oxygenation or an admixture of venous blood occurs centrally in the heart or lungs. In the heart it is produced by a shunt of venous blood from the right side to the left through a congenital communication. In the lungs it may be due to the passage of blood through unaerated alveoli. Central cyanosis is characteristically seen in warm parts and is best assessed in the tongue which is also the most reliable guide to the haemoglobin content of the blood. By contrast, peripheral cyanosis occurs in cold extremities where arteriolar constriction and capillary dilatation have resulted in slowing of the blood flow and increased formation of reduced haemoglobin. Peripheral cyanosis is serious if the constriction is due to a low cardiac output and the malar flush of mitral stenosis or myxoedema is an example of this. Frequently, however, peripheral cyanosis occurs independently of heart disease. It may be simply a normal response to cold or abnormal activity of the arterioles as in Raynaud's phenomenon.

The thyroid gland

Thyroid disease is an important and frequently overlooked cause of heart disease. To palpate the gland the physician should stand *behind* the patient who is given water to swallow when asked. Movement of the lobes and isthmus can then be readily detected and the presence of enlargement or nodules noted. Bruits over the gland must be sought and distinguished from those arising in the heart or neck vessels. The fine tremor of thyrotoxicosis is best demonstrated by placing a small sheet of paper or thin card on the dorsum of the outpsread fingers and the temperature of the hands and texture of the hair and skin are vital clues. Eye signs are relatively uncommon compared with other symptoms and signs and thinning of the outer third of the eyebrows occurs normally with age.

The jugular venous pressure

This is best assessed by studying the pulsations of the *internal* jugular vein. These are invariably discoverable provided that the superior vena cava is patent. By contrast the external veins are frequently invisible; when visible they are commonly obstructed, and when both visible and unobstructed they are misleading. They should therefore be disregarded. Students often find difficulty at first in recognising internal jugular pulsation and the following method is suggested to assist them to gain confidence. A line (AB) is drawn in washable ink from the clavicle 2 cm lateral to the sterno-clavicular joint, to the mastoid process. This marks the course of the internal jugular vein. The line is then intersected by a series of short lines at right angles to it (Fig. 2.2). If the neck is now inspected from a position in front of the patient the intersections will be seen to show an undulatory movement. The highest shows the upper limit of the internal jugular pulsations which are made more easily visible by the ink lines. If the patient is asked to sit more upright, a lower intersection will be found to move, and if he lies flat a higher intersection shows the characteristic undulation. If the patient is wearing a necklace, its chain can be moved to various positions of the neck to act as an alternative marker of the pulsations. The venous pressure is measured in centimetres of blood by noting the vertical height at which the pulsations are seen above the horizontal level of the sternal angle. The observer's fist placed on the sternal angle forms a convenient measure, for the knuckles are approximately 1, 3, 5 and 7 centimetres above it (Fig. 2.2). Normally the pressure ranges from 0 to 2 cm vertically above the sternal angle when the patient lies at 45°. Although it is customary to measure it with the patient semi-recumbent with his trunk at 45° to the horizontal, the *vertical height* of the pulsation above the sternal angle and hence the venous pressure varies very little with change of posture. If the pressure is low, pulsations may be visible only in the supine position, while a very high pressure produces tense veins and small amplitude pulsations which only become evident when the patient sits bolt upright or stands.

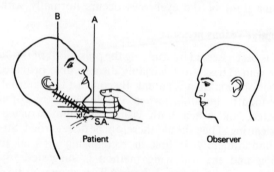

Fig. 2.2 Clinical measurement of the jugular venous pressure. AB represent an ink-line drawn from a point 3-finger-breadths lateral to the sterno-clavicular joint (the surface marking of the jugular bulb) to the mastoid process; it is intersected by a series of short transverse lines X, X_1, etc. The patient is observed frontally to find the uppermost intersection which shows an undulatory movement. The level of this above the sternal angle is measured with the physician's fist placed on the sternal angle (S–A). The knuckles measure approximately 1, 3, 5 and 7 cm. The pressure is normally 0–2 cm above the sternal angle.

In sinus rhythm, venous pulsation has an undulatory character (Fig. 2.3a) and in atrial fibrillation it shows a large amplitude systolic wave synchronous with the carotid pulse (Fig. 2.3d) which is palpated with the thumb on the other side of the neck (Fig 2.4). These characteristics usually serve to identify venous pulsation with ease but the following additional features may be helpful to the beginner. It is usually impalpable, varies in height and amplitude with posture and respiration and is abolished by relatively light

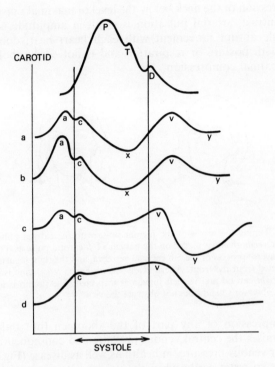

Fig. 2.3 The jugular venous pulse. The arterial pulse is used to time events in the venous pulse. (a) The normal venous pulse. The 'a' wave is caused by the rise of pressure due to atrial contraction. The pressure then falls as the atrium relaxes producing the 'x' descent interrupted momentarily by the 'c' wave which marks tricuspid closure. Thus the jugular pulse characteristically *falls* in systole as the arterial pulse *rises*. The pressure then rises as the atrium fills until the tricuspid valve opens at the apex of v when it falls again (y). (b) Giant 'a' waves. These are seen as abrupt 'flicking' waves resembling the arterial pulse in quality but preceding it in time. They occur if there is obstruction to outflow from the right atrium due to tricuspid stenosis or right ventricular hypertrophy. The hypertrophic ventricle has a reduced compliance and requires a powerful atrial contraction to distend it. The hypertrophy may be due to pulmonary stenosis or pulmonary hypertension. (c) The pulse in pericardial disease and restrictive cardiomyopathy. The contour is dominated by the sharp 'y' descent. The other waves are small and the pressure is found to be high. (d) The venous pulse in atrial fibrillation. In the absence of atrial contraction, 'a' and 'x' waves do not occur and the pulse *rises* in systole (cv).

compression of the neck below the level of maximal pulsation. By contrast, arterial pulsation is small in amplitude, shows a single abrupt movement with each heart beat, does not vary with posture or respiration and is not easily abolished by proximal compression.

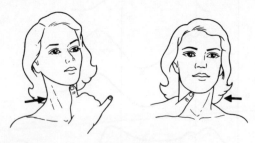

Fig. 2.4 Timing .the waves of the jugular pulse with the carotid pulse. The observer's *right thumb* is placed on the patient's *left* carotid pulse as it crosses the transverse process of the 5th cervical vertebra, and the right jugular pulse is inspected from the front. Alternatively the observers *left* thumb is placed on the *right* carotid and the left jugular is inspected. The thumb is used so that the observer's hand does not obstruct the view.

Compression of any part of the abdomen (not only the liver) raises the central venous pressure and consequently the jugular venous pressure, in health as well as disease (Fig. 2.5). It does so more easily when the venous pressure and blood volume are increased as in heart failure but the manoeuvre

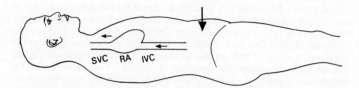

Fig. 2.5 Abdominal compression and the jugular venous pressure. Compression of any part of the abdomen raises the pressure in the inferior vena cava (IVC). Unless the IVC is completely obstructed the rise in pressure is transmitted to the right atrium (RA) and the superior vena cava (SVC). There is *no* reflux from the liver to the jugular vein (no 'hepato-jugular reflux'). The increase in jugular pressure occurs in normal subjects but it is more obvious if there is an increased blood volume or the venous pressure is already raised.

gives no more information than can be derived from the procedures already described and there is no such thing as 'hepato-jugular reflux' or 'reflex'.

The jugular venous pulse

The pulse is next inspected for abnormalities of contour. Normally there are three positive waves, a, c and v, and two negative waves, x and y (Fig. 2.3a). The 'a' wave is produced by a rise of pressure due to atrial systole and the succeeding negative wave 'x' by the fall of pressure caused by atrial relaxation. The 'x' descent is momentarily interrupted by the 'c' wave which is a carotid artefact. Pulsation may be produced partly by tricuspid closure and partly by transmission of the carotid pulse. Blood continues to flow into the atrium during atrial relaxation and since the tricuspid valve is closed, the atrial pressure begins to rise again producing the 'v' wave. When the tricuspid valve opens in early diastole the atrial pressure falls producing the 'y' dip. Several important abnormalities of the venous pulse can be recognized.

1. *Exaggerated 'a' waves*
These occur when there is an impediment to the passage of blood from the atrium to the ventricle. If the right ventricle is hypertrophied, it is relatively uncompliant and the atrium has to contract unduly forcefully to distend it. Giant 'a' waves are therefore found in pulmonary hypertension and pulmonary stenosis. Tricuspid stenosis acts as a more direct obstruction and similarly causes exaggerated 'a' waves. The waves are timed by placing a thumb on the carotid artery on the opposite side of the neck. Giant 'a' waves appear as a sudden, transient, flicking pulsation which at first glance may be mistaken for arterial pulsation. Timing the waves, however, with the carotid pulse prevents this error (Figs. 2.3b and 2.4).

2. *Atrial fibrillation and tricuspid reflux*
In atrial fibrillation the 'a' and 'x' waves, due respectively to atrial contraction and relaxation, are absent and the jugular pulse shows only 'c', 'v' and 'y' waves. The absence of the 'x' trough causes the pulse to show a systolic expansion synchronous with carotid pulsation (Fig. 2.3d). It remains

easy, however, to distinguish it from arterial pulsation by its leisurely expansion and relatively large amplitude; this systolic expansion of the venous pulse was described by Mackenzie in 1896 and is diagnostic of atrial fibrillation. When tricuspid reflux is associated with atrial fibrillation the venous pulse has the same wave form but a much larger amplitude. Tricuspid reflux with sinus rhythm does not produce an abnormality of the wave-form recognisable at the bedside.

3. *Exaggerated 'y' trough*

When the venous pressure is extremely high, as in constrictive pericarditis, cardiomyopathy and occasionally in congestive heart failure due to commoner causes, the amplitude of the 'a', 'c' and 'v' waves may be very small and the undulations of the venous pulse may be dominated by a sudden deep 'y' wave in diastole (Fig. 2.3c).

4. *Cannon waves*

If the atrium contracts when the tricuspid valve is closed, (i.e. during ventricular systole), a jet of blood is forced into the jugular veins and a visible 'cannon' wave results (Fig. 2.6). Such simultaneous atrial and ventricular contractions occur irregularly in the presence of atrial or ventricular ectopic beats, heart block or ventricular tachycardia. In the latter two conditions *irregular* cannon waves contrast with the *regular* heart action. In nodal rhythm however, the P wave regularly accompanies or follows the QRS and atrial contraction always occurs during ventricular systole; the resulting cannon waves are therefore *regular* and synchronous with heart beat at 40 to 60 per minute.

Palpation of the heart

This is one of the most informative procedures in clinical cardiology because it is often the most reliable method of answering the crucial question, 'is the heart enlarged and if so which ventricle is involved?' It must, therefore, be practised with great care and patience.

The apex beat

This is the most infero-lateral point on the left side of the chest at which the cardiac impulse can be *distinctly* felt. Normally the apex beat is in the 5th space within the mid-clavicular line. The position of the apex beat should be expressed in terms of its relation to the intercostal spaces and the mid-clavicular, anterior axillary, mid-axillary and posterior axillary lines. It is normally in the 5th space (sometimes 4th in children) within the mid-clavicular line.

The quality of the apical impulse. Normally the apex beat is produced by the pointed tip of the left ventricle. It is this shape which produces the characteristic gently thrusting quality of the normal apical impulse which is confined to a circular area about 2 cm in diameter.

If the cardiac impulse is felt to the left of the mid-clavicular line this may be due either to displacement of the heart by lung disease or scoliosis or to cardiac hypertrophy. In the latter case the quality of the cardiac impulse will be abnormal and indicate left or right ventricular hypertrophy or both.

Left ventricular hypertrophy. In left ventricular hypertrophy, the thrust is exaggerated and it may be described as heaving

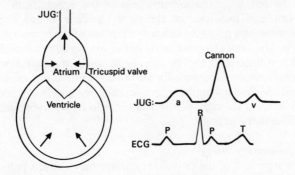

Fig. 2.6 The mode of production of 'cannon' waves. If a 'P' wave occurs during ventricular systole, due either to an ectopic beat or heart block, atrial contraction occurs when the tricuspid valve is closed by ventricular contraction, and the rise of atrial pressure is transmitted to the jugular vein as an abrupt wave or 'cannon' wave. If atrial and ventricular contractions occur independently as in ectopic beats, heart block or ventricular tachycardia, the 'cannon' waves are irregular; in nodal rhythm the 'P' wave regularly accompanies or follows the QRS and the 'cannon' waves therefore occur regularly with each heart beat, at a rate of 20–40 per minute in adults, or up to 60 per minute in children.

but the area of the impulse remains relatively small and is often a circle of no more than 3–4 cm diameter. The heart may cause an adjacent rib to move and this is a reliable sign of cardiac hypertrophy regardless of the position of the impulse.

Right ventricular hypertrophy. The anterior surface of the right ventricle has a gently curving convex surface and has no pointed area comparable to the apex of the left ventricle. When it is enlarged it therefore gives a diffuse impulse which may be transmitted to an area several centimetres wide, and may be felt as far as the apical region. If the first heart sound is accentuated, as in mitral stenosis, it may be palpable and this together with the diffuse pulsation, imparts a 'tapping' sensation to the hand. An enlarged right ventricle may also produce a palpable thrust in the third and fourth left interspaces close to the sternum and may even produce movement of the sternum itself. When right ventricular hypertrophy is caused by emphysema this sign is obscured by the intervening voluminous lung but the hypertrophied right ventricle can then be felt by palpating upwards in the epigastrium. The amplitude of pulsation of the right ventricle in any one of these three sites may give a clue to the cause of the hypertrophy. A large amplitude (hyperkinetic impulse) suggests an increased stroke volume and the possibility of valve regurgitation or a shunt; while a powerfully sustained contraction of small amplitude (hyperdynamic impulse) suggests an obstruction to outflow from the right ventricle as in pulmonary hypertension or pulmonary stenosis.

The pulmonary artery

Enlargement of the pulmonary artery may cause a palpable thrust in the second left interspace close to the sternum.

The aorta

Enlargement of the aorta is only palpable when due to an aneurysm which produces pulsation most often in the second intercostal space but occasionally elsewhere on the anterior chest. Arterial pulsation in the suprasternal notch is due to an abnormally high aortic arch. In adults this may be caused (especially in women) by obesity with high diaphragms, but in children and young adults it is pathognomonic of coarctation of the aorta.

Kinked carotid artery

With the development of obesity and high diaphragms in women, the *right* common carotid artery may become too long for the course it has to run; it becomes folded upon itself producing a pulsatile swelling a little smaller than a cherry in the lower third of the right side of the neck (Fig. 2.7) which is commonly mistaken for an aneurysm of the carotid artery.

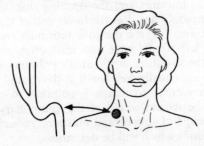

Fig. 2.7 A kinked carotid artery produces a pulsatile swelling a little smaller than a cherry in the course of the right common carotid artery in the lower third of the neck of obese women.

Percussion

This technique is of no value in determining heart size. Two points about it however, are worth considering. Absence of cardiac dullness may be due to over-distension of the lungs as in emphysema, and dullness in the second intercostal space suggests the possibility of an aneurysm of the aorta or enlargement of the pulmonary artery amongst possible causes.

Auscultation

It is essential to use a correctly designed stethoscope and students should beware of the innumerable poorly designed and ill-conceived instruments available. In the writer's opinion the best instrument is the Littman stethoscope which combines acoustic excellence with elegance of design and comfort in use.

In the description of sounds and murmurs which follows, it will be noted that positions on the chest are referred to in anatomical terms. The use of such expressions as 'the mitral area' 'the tricuspid area' etc., which is unfortunately common, is to be avoided. The premises upon which such terms are based are fallacious and the use of them leads to innumerable mistakes for the following reasons.

Murmurs due to aortic valve disease are often heard at the apex, which is commonly referred to as the 'mitral area' and therefore erroneously supposed to be due to mitral disease; mitral systolic murmurs and the opening snap of the mitral valve are commonly heard at the lower end of the sternum— the 'tricuspid area'. Aortic diastolic murmurs are most often heard at the left sternal edge and least often at the second right space, the so-called 'aortic area'. Pulmonary and aortic valve closure are equally well heard at the second left space— the 'pulmonary area', so that it is pointless to compare the intensity of the second sound at the 'pulmonary and aortic areas'. The origin of sounds and murmurs should be decided on other grounds which will be described.

The first heart sound

This is a low-pitched, dull sound best heard at the apex and lower sternum; it has two components thought to be produced by mitral and tricuspid valve closure in that order, and these may be incompletely fused so that splitting may be audible (Fig. 2.8). The loudness of the sound is not a reliable guide to the strength of ventricular contraction and depends almost entirely upon the degree of opening of the A–V valves at the moment of ventricular contraction, which in turn depends on the P–R interval. If this is optimal, between 0.12–0.18 sec., atrial contraction opens the A–V valves fully just before ventricular contraction which then closes them with the production of a loud sound. If the interval is either longer or shorter than this the valves are not fully open and ventricular contraction produces only a quiet sound or even no sound at all (Fig. 2.9).

In mitral valve disease the first sound may be characteristically accentuated due to sudden tension of the fused thickened cusps in mitral stenosis or quiet or even absent if the valve is so diseased that it cannot close in mitral regurgitation.

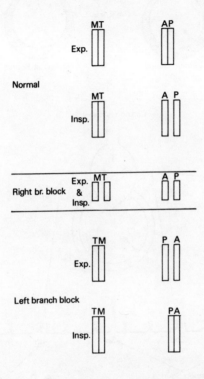

Fig. 2.8 The first and second heart sounds. M and T represent closure of the mitral and tricuspid valves respectively. P and A represent pulmonary and aortic closure. Inspiration delays pulmonary valve closure mainly by increasing the filling of the right heart. In right bundle branch block tricuspid and pulmonary closure are delayed in all phases of respiraton and there is 'fixed' splitting of the first and second sounds. In left bundle branch block, aortic valve closure is constantly delayed and follows pulmonary closure. The latter is delayed in the normal fashion by inspiration so that the split may paradoxically disappear in that phase of respiration.

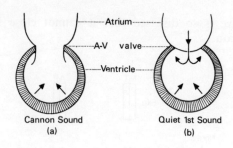

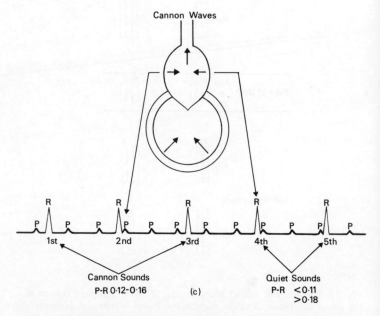

Fig. 2.9 The variation in intensity of the first heart sound in atrio-ventricular block. The loudest ('cannon') sounds occur when the a–v valves are widest open at the moment of ventricular contraction (a). This is the case when atrial contraction occurs about 0.12–0.16 sec before ventricular contraction. If the P–R interval is shorter than this, atrial contraction cannot open the valve fully before ventricular contraction occurs; if it is longer, the valve cusps float into the closed position on the rising tide of blood entering the ventricle (b). In either case the valve is almost closed when the ventricle contracts and a quiet sound results. It will be noted that the 'cannon' waves of the jugular pulse previously described, do not coincide with 'cannon' sounds. They occur in cardiac cycles having *quiet* heart sounds (c).

The second heart sound

This is sharper in quality than the first sound and can be heard all over the precordium. It is best analysed, however, at the second and third interspaces close to the sternum. If the student practices auscultation in children or young adults, he will find that the second heart sound at these positions is single in expiration but becomes split on inspiration. The first component of the split is produced by aortic valve closure and the second by pulmonary valve closure (Fig. 2.8) and inspiration causes splitting by delaying the pulmonary component. This normal splitting of the second heart sound is of the utmost value in bedside diagnosis. It enables differentiation of extra-cardiac or 'innocent' childhood murmurs from those due to atrial septal defect or pulmonary stenosis. In the former conditions the second sound splits normally but in the latter there is persistent wide separation of the two components. The loudness of the pulmonary component is a rather poor guide to the pulmonary artery pressure but the degree of separation of the components is a quite good guide to the severity of atrial septal defect or pulmonary stenosis.

If activation of the left ventricle is delayed as in left bundle branch block, the relationship of aortic to pulmonary valve closure is reversed and the pulmonary component preceeds the aortic. Inspiration then has a paradoxical effect, the second sound becoming single in inspiration and splitting in expiration (Fig. 2.8).

The third heart sound

This is a dull, low-pitched, quiet sound, following closely upon the second sound in early diastole and may be caused either by a movement of the A–V valves or vibration of the ventricular wall in the rapid filling phase (Fig. 2.10). It is best heard at the lower sternum if it comes from the right heart, at the apex if it comes from the left ventricle. It is normally heard in children and young adults but becomes progressively less common with age and is usually pathological if heard in subjects over the age of 35. It occurs in conditions associated with a large stroke volume and rapid ventricular filling, such as ventricular septal defect and mitral reflux, but it also occurs in left ventricular failure due to hypertension or cardiac infarction.

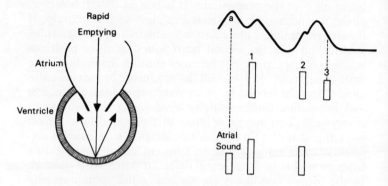

Fig. 2.10 The third heart sound and the atrial (4th) sound. Both of these sounds occur during periods of rapid ventricular filling. The atrial sound coincides with the accelerated filling produced by atrial contraction. The third heart sound occurs during the rapid filling phase in early diastole when the rapidly falling intraventricular pressure momentarily drops below the atrial pressure which has mounted during the preceding ventricular systole.

The fourth heart sound

This resembles the third heart sound in quality and the sites at which it is heard, but occurs in the rapid filling phase of presystole just before the first heart sound (Fig. 2.10). In fact it is often confused with splitting of the first heart sound. The latter, however, produces two components of equal sharpness whereas a fourth sound is duller than the succeeding first heart sound, resembling 'lul-lub-dup' (4th, 1st–2nd), and may be made inaudible by firm pressure with the stethoscope. It is due to atrial contraction and cannot, therefore, occur in atrial fibrillation. Although it can be recorded phono-cardiographically in normal subjects, it is only heard with the ordinary stethoscope in pathological conditions when the atria are contracting unduly forcefully to fill a hypertrophied, and therefore uncompliant, ventricle. It also occurs if the ventricle is damaged as in ischaemic heart disease; then a more powerful atrial contraction produces a higher presystolic pressure in the ventricle, increased stretch of the ventricular muscle and by Starling's law, increased force of contraction of the remaining healthy muscle, so that a normal output can be maintained. For the same reasons it can be heard during an attack of angina when the ventricular muscle is working inefficiently owing to transient ischaemia.

Triple rhythm and gallop rhythm

The term triple rhythm is used to describe the presence of three heart sounds in each heart cycle due to the addition of the third or fourth sounds previously described. It is better to avoid the use of this term and to say which additional sound is present if it can be accurately timed. This may be difficult if there is tachycardia, when the presence of third or fourth heart sounds may produce a cadence resembling that of a galloping horse. The term 'gallop-rhythm' is then useful and appropriate. In tachycardia, diastole may be so shortened that the third and fourth sounds become synchronous and a 'summation gallop' is produced.

Ejection click

This is a sharp sound occurring very early in systole and best heard at the base of the heart (Fig. 2.11a). It is frequently mistaken for the first heart sound, but this error will not be made if it is remembered that the first sound is best heard at the apex or lower sternum. If an early systolic sound is heard more sharply at the base than the apex, it is likely to be an ejection click produced by the sudden tension of the walls of a dilated pulmonary artery or aorta as the blood is ejected into it. It occurs in conditions causing dilatation of the aorta or pulmonary artery, such as patent ductus arteriosus or atrial septal defect, and idiopathic dilatation of the pulmonary artery. It may also occur in pulmonary or aortic stenosis when it is due to tension of the fused cusps.

Other systolic clicks

A mid-systolic click often followed by a murmur may occur in non-rheumatic mitral reflux (Fig. 2.11b). The click may then be mistaken for the second heart sound, and the late systolic murmur which follows it is erroneously supposed to be diastolic in time. Careful auscultation and comparison with the sounds at other sites will prevent this mistake. Systolic clicks also occur if there is a small pneumothorax, or following pericarditis.

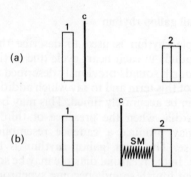

Fig. 2.11 Systolic clicks. (a) An ejection click (c) occurs in early systole and coincides with the abrupt rise in pressure in a dilated aorta or pulmonary artery. Aortic ejection clicks occur in patent ductus arteriosus, in the post-stenotic dilatation of aortic stenosis and also with a bicuspid valve. Pulmonary ejection clicks occur in idiopathic dilatation of the pulmonary artery, pulmonary hypertension and the post-stenotic dilatation of pulmonary stenosis. (b) A mid-systolic click (c) followed by a systolic murmur (SM). This is due to a congenital anomaly of one of the chordae or of the posterior cusp of the mitral valve. In either case the cusp becomes taut as it balloons into the atrium and some regurgitation follows.

Mid-systolic murmurs

Figure 2.12 shows that there is an appreciable interval between the first heart sound and the moment when ejection of blood into the aorta occurs with consequent equalization of aortic and intraventricular pressures. There must, therefore, be a similar interval between the first heart sound and the beginning of a murmur due to passage of blood from the ventricles into the great vessels. Such a murmur will grow in intensity to a peak in mid-systole and thereafter wane and cease before the second heart sound. It is this latter feature which enables recognition of mid-systolic murmurs at the

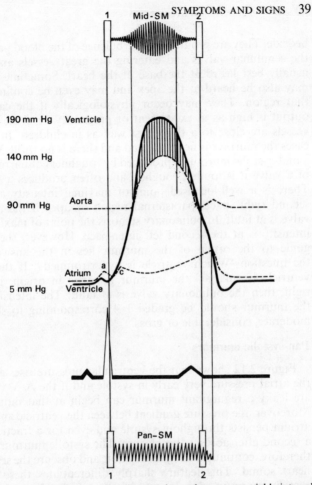

Fig. 2.12 Systolic murmurs. The diagram shows that an appreciable interval occurs between the first heart sound (1) and the moment when the ventricular pressure (solid line) equals the aortic diastolic pressure (upper broken line). A murmur (mid-SM) due to ejection of blood from ventricle to aorta (or pulmonary artery) cannot begin earlier than this. It waxes in intensity to mid-systole and then wanes as ejection diminishes with the falling intra-ventricular pressure. By contrast the ventricular pressure has to rise only a little to exceed the atrial pressure so that the time interval between the first sound and a murmur due to reflux through the a–v valves may be negligible. The pressure gradient between atrium and ventricle persists after the second sound (2) so that the murmur is pan-systolic (Pan-SM) and may even be prolonged into early diastole.

bedside. They are produced by turbulence of the blood passing the semilunar valves and entering the great vessels and are usually best heard at the base of the heart. Sometimes they may also be heard at the apex and may even be confined to that region. They may occur physiologically if the cardiac output is high as in excitement or pregnancy or if the great vessels are close to a thin chest wall as in children. In such cases the murmur is not very loud and there is no thrill. When a mid-systolic murmur is produced by roughness or narrowing of a valve it is louder, rougher, and often produces a thrill. There is a well-localised point of maximal intensity at the second right space, parasternal region or apex if the aortic valve is at fault. In pulmonary stenosis the point of maximum intensity is at the second left interspace. However, the best guide to the origin of the murmur lies in the answer to the question 'Which ventricle is hypertrophied?' If the left ventricle is enlarged the murmur is aortic in origin; if the right, then the pulmonary valve is at fault. The intensity of the murmur should be graded 1–4 corresponding to slight, moderate, considerable or gross.

Pan-systolic murmurs

Figure 2.12 shows that the ventricular pressure rises above the atrial pressure very early in systole and if the A–V valves are leaky a regurgitant murmur can begin at that moment. Moreover, the pressure gradient between the ventricle and the atrium persists throughout systole and even for a fraction of a second after aortic valve closure. The systolic murmur can, therefore, continue throughout systole and obscure the second heart sound. This feature sharply differentiates these *pan-systolic* murmurs due to regurgitation from those due to ejection through the semilunar valves which cease before the second sound. Pan-systolic murmurs often have a 'blowing' character, but they may be musical or even have a 'seagull' quality. Mitral regurgitant murmurs are usually best heard at the apex and radiate towards the axilla; but it is interesting that those due to a leaking mitral prosthesis are best heard over the surface marking of the valve and prosthesis at the lower end of the sternum, where murmurs due to tricuspid regurgitation are also heard best. A mitral regurgitant murmur

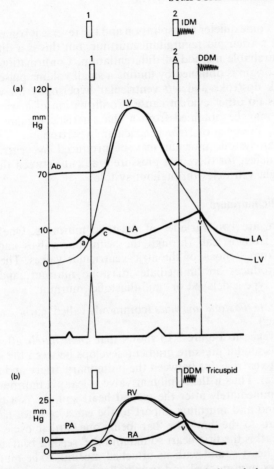

Fig. 2.13 Diastolic murmurs. A murmur due to a leak through the semilunar valves occurs *immediately* (IDM) following the second sound, because there is an *immediate* pressure gradient. Following the second sound there is an interval until the ventricular and atrial pressures equalize and the a–v valves open. There is therefore a *delay* between the second sound and the beginning of murmurs originating in these valves. They are therefore called 'delayed' diastolic murmurs (DDM). The delay is longer in mitral than in tricuspid murmurs because the left ventricular pressure must fall 60 mm Hg to equalize with the left atrial pressure, but the right ventricular pressure has to full only about 10 mmHg to reach the right atrial pressure. (LV = Left Ventricle. Ao = Aorta: LA = Left Atrium: PA = Pulmonary Artery: RV = Right Ventricle: RA = Right Atrium.

may become quieter in inspiration and the reverse is sometimes true of a tricuspid regurgitant murmur, but this is a difficult and unreliable method of differentiation. Confirmation of a mitral origin is obtained by finding a small volume pulse with a quick upstroke and *left* ventricular hypertophy for which there is no other evident cause. Confirmation of a tricuspid origin may be obtained from a characteristic jugular pulse and the presence of *right* ventricular hypertrophy.

A pan-systolic murmur may be produced by ventricular septal defect for there is a pressure gradient between the left and right ventricles throughout systole.

Diastolic murmurs

There are two varieties of diastolic murmurs. One type results from a leak through the semilunar valves and the other from stenosis of the atrio-ventricular valves. The first type produces an 'immediate' diastolic murmur, and the second type a delayed or 'mid-diastolic' murmur.

Immediate diastolic murmurs (commonly called 'early diastolic')

Reference to Figure 2.13 shows that *immediately* after the second sound a pressure gradient develops between the aorta and left ventricle (or between the pulmonary artery and right ventricle). Thus if the semilunar valve is leaky a murmur can begin immediately after the second heart sound. As a result the sound and murmurs impart to the ear a cadence having two beats to the 'bar', the 'bar' being one cardiac cycle. The 'first beat' is the first heart sound and the 'second beat' is the second heart sound with its attached murmur. The murmur is always high pitched and usually diminuendo in quality. It is beat heard with the diaphragm of the stethoscope with the patient upright and leaning forward holding his breath in full expiration. Whether due to aortic or pulmonary reflux the murmurs are most often heard at the left parasternal region and only exceptionally is the murmur of aortic reflux best heard at the second right space or the apex. As usual the decision as to which valve is producing the murmur depends on the presence or absence of confirmatory signs. Pulmonary reflux should only be diagnosed when there is clear clinical evidence of *gross* right ventricular hypertrophy; but it is quite safe to attribute an early diastolic murmur to aortic reflux even in the absence of left ventricular hypertrophy or confirmatory signs in the pulse, though the lesion must then be mild.

Delayed diastolic murmurs (commonly called 'mid-diastolic')

Reference to Figure 2.13 shows that there is an appreciable interval between the second heart sound produced by aortic valve closure and the moment when the ventricular pressures have fallen below the atrial pressure with consequent opening of the A–V valves. A murmur derived from the A–V valves cannot therefore begin during this interval and the ear will detect a cadence with 'three beats to the bar'. The first 'beat' is the first heart sound, the second is the second heart sound and after a brief delay, the third 'beat', which is the *delayed* diastolic murmur, is heard. This delay alone serves to differentiate these murmurs from the immediate diastolic murmurs previously described but there are further differentiating features. If due to mitral stenosis, the murmur is low-pitched, rumbling and usually localised to a small area at or lateral to the apex. Like all sounds originating in the mitral valve or left ventricle it is best heard with the patient in the left lateral position. The duration of the murmur should be graded when the heart rate is 70–80/min.

It may be so short as to simulate a third heart sound (Grade 1) or so long as to fill diastole to the succeeding first heart sound (Grade 4); or it may be of intermediate duration (Grade 2 or 3). If there is atrial fibrillation the duration should be noted in the longer cardiac cycles. Tricuspid diastolic murmurs are best heard at the lower end of the sternum. Figure 2.13b shows that the beginning of the murmur is only very slightly delayed after the second sound since the pressure has only to fall from the pulmonary diastolic pressure of about 20 to a raised right atrial pressure in tricuspid stenosis of about 10 mmHg. Nevertheless a three-beat cadence can usually be detected.

The Graham Steell murmur

This murmur was first described as the murmur of pulmonary

hypertension in cases of mitral stenosis. It is an immediate diastolic murmur due to pulmonary reflux. The murmur is relatively uncommon and should be diagnosed only if there is evidence of *gross* right ventricular hypertrophy. If this is lacking, immediate diastolic murmurs at the left sternal edge should always be attributed to aortic reflux, even in the absence of confirmatory signs.

The Austin Flint murmur

This eponymous title refers to a murmur which exactly resembles that of mitral stenosis but occurs in patients with *gross* aortic reflux, usually syphilitic. It is thought to be due to the regurgitant jet from the leaky aortic valve striking the adjacent cusp of the mitral valve and causing partial closure. This narrowing of the mitral orifice naturally results in a murmur having precisely similar characteristics to those of organic mitral stenosis. The diagnosis of an Austin Flint murmur should only be made if there is evidence of *gross* aortic reflux with conspicuous left ventricular hypertrophy and a water-hammer pulse.

Continuous murmurs

These are continuous from one first sound to the next and, therefore, continue through the second heart sound. The following are the main varieties:

Venous hum
Patent ductus arteriosus
Subclavian-pulmonary anastomosis (Blalock Operation)
Enlarged breast arteries in pregnancy
Enlarged bronchial arteries in pulmonary atresia
Abnormal coronary artery communicating with right heart
Ruptured sinus of Valsalva
Arteriovenous aneurysm of the lung

The venous hum is by far the commonest of these and can be detected in many children over the manubrium sterni or below the clavicles. It commonly changes in quality and intensity from systole to diastole but it is usually relatively quiet and never accompanied by a thrill. It can always be abolished or accentuated by altering the position of the head or compressing the jugular bulb or internal jugular vein and although its characteristics make it easy to recognize, it is often confused with murmurs of organic origin.

FURTHER READING

Leatham, Aubrey (1975) *Auscultation of the heart and Phonocardiography* Edinburgh: Churchill Livingstone.

Symposium (1971) Pathophysiology and Differential Diagnosis (Symptoms and Signs). *Progress in Cardiovascular Disease*, **13**, no. 6 and **14**, nos. 1 and 2.

3. Haemodynamics

With the introduction of cardiac catheterization and of needle puncture of the various cardiac chambers into clinical practice, it has become possible to obtain blood samples and pressure measurements from all four cardiac chambers, and to assess disturbances of the circulation quantitatively. This has so greatly increased our knowledge of the correlation of patho-physiology with symptoms and signs that in some cases the use of these techniques is now redundant. This is often true in the selection of cases of mitral or aortic stenosis for operative treatment, but in complicated disorders the information given by these methods is indispensable for a thorough appraisal. In the following section the kind of information which can be obtained from these investigations will be defined and a brief account given of the nature, risks and indications for the various procedures.

Four parameters can be studied, namely *Flow, Pressure, Resistance* and *Pressure Pulse* contours.

Flow—The cardiac output

The cardiac output is estimated by application of the Fick principle which states that:

$$\text{Cardiac output (l/min)} = \frac{\text{Oxygen consumption (ml/min)}}{\text{Arterio-venous oxygen difference (ml/l)}}$$

It will be seen that the denominator of this equation indicates the amount of oxygen each litre of blood has taken up in the lungs and if the amount of oxygen consumed per minute is divided by this value, the dividend indicates the number of litres of blood which has passed through the lungs in one minute.

The oxygen consumption is measured either by spirometry or the Douglas bag method. In order to obtain the oxygen saturation of blood reaching the lungs it is essential to obtain a thoroughly mixed sample, because samples of blood returned from the limbs, brain and viscera differ in oxygen content. Mixing is only complete when the blood reaches the right ventricle or pulmonary artery and a sample from the latter is the most desirable. For practical purposes brachial or femoral arterial oxygen saturation can be assumed to represent the saturation of blood leaving the lungs.

Pressure

If the cardiac catheter is connected to a suitable electro-manometer, a graphic record can be made of the pressure pulse from the various cardiac chambers and systolic, diastolic and mean pressures can be measured. Zero is taken as the point 10 cm anterior to the skin of the back. Normal values are as follows:

R.A. (mean) 0–5 mmHg   L.A. mean = 5–12 mmHg

R.V. $\frac{15-30}{0-5}$ mmHg   L.V. $\frac{100-150}{0-10}$ mmHg

P.A. $\frac{15-30}{5-15}$ mmHg   (mean 10 − 20mmHg)

Resistance

The resistance in a hydraulic circuit is given by Poiseuille's equation which states:

$$\text{Resistance (R)} = \frac{\text{Pressure (P) Gradient}}{\text{Flow (F)}}$$

therefore,

The Pulmonary Vascular Resistance (P.V.R.) =

$$\frac{\text{P.A.Pm—L.A.Pm (mmHg)}}{\text{Pulmonary Blood Flow (l/min)}}$$

where P.A.Pm and L.A.Pm are the mean pulmonary artery and left atrial pressures respectively.

The P.V.R. is expressed in units derived directly from the formula and arbitrarily graded, as described by Wood. Substituting normal values we might have

$$\text{P.V.R.} = \frac{12-6 \text{ mmHg}}{6 l/min} = 1 \text{ Unit}$$

The normal P.V.R. is less than 2 units. A resistance between 2 and 5 units may be regarded as slightly raised; between 5 and 8 units moderately raised; between 8 and 10 units considerably raised and over 10 units grossly raised.

The Systemic Resistance =

$$\frac{\text{Mean Arterial—Mean Venous Pressure (mmHg)}}{\text{Systemic Flow (l/min)}}$$

The normal systemic resistance lies between 10 and 20 units.

The relationships between pressure, flow and resistance

Consideration of the above formulae shows that pressure, flow and resistance are always inter-related and it is meaningless to consider any one of them in isolation.

Example 1

$$\text{P.V.R.} = \frac{30\text{–}6 \text{ mmHg)}}{12 \text{ l/Min}} = 2 \text{ Units}$$

The output is greatly raised but the pulmonary artery mean pressure of 30 mm Hg is elevated proportionately, simply due to the increased flow and the resistance is normal. This is called *hyperkinetic pulmonary hypertension*.

Example 2

$$\text{P.V.R.} = \frac{46\text{–}6 \text{ mmHg}}{4 \text{ l/Min}} = 10 \text{ Units}$$

The pulmonary artery mean pressure is greatly raised, the left atrial pressure is normal and the flow is reduced. The high resistance is due to narrowing of the pulmonary arterioles.

Example 3

$$\text{P.V.R.} = \frac{25\text{–}15 \text{ mmHg}}{5 \text{ l/Min}} = 2 \text{ Units}$$

The left atrial pressure is raised and the pulmonary artery pressure is raised proportionately. The flow is normal. This may occur in the early stages of mitral stenosis before narrowing of the pulmonary arterioles occurs. Later in the disease a disproportionate rise of the pulmonary artery pressure occurs and the resistance is increased owing to arteriolar narrowing.

Example 4

$$\text{P.V.R.} = \frac{78\text{–}6 \text{ mmHg}}{12 \text{ l/Min}} = 6 \text{ Units}$$

The left atrial pressure is normal but the pulmonary artery pressure and flow are increased and so is the resistance. This might be found in congenital heart disease with a left to right shunt. Closure of the defect would reduce the flow to normal but the raised resistance shows that the raised pulmonary artery pressure is partly due to arteriolar narrowing and the pressure might not return to normal.

Pressure gradients

An obstruction in the circulation whether it is gradual or abrupt causes a pressure difference or *gradient* across it. For example, the resistance offered by arterioles causes the pressure in large vessels such as the aorta or femoral artery to exceed that in the capillaries. The pressure gradient occurs gradually in the arterioles. However, if there is an abrupt obstruction, as by a narrowed valve, there is an abrupt pressure change across it; the magnitude of the gradient is proportional to the *blood flow* and to the *resistance* offered by the obstruction. The same principles, therefore, govern the relationships between pressure, flow and resistance as have already been described. The severity of the obstruction can be assessed only if both the pressure gradient and flow are known.

It is possible to measure the pressure gradient across each of the four heart valves and by relating it to flow, to assess the degree of narrowing of a diseased or abnormal valve.

Pressure pulse contours

The pressure pulses recorded by electro-manometers from each of the cardiac chambers and from the great vessels have characteristic contours, and abnormalities of these may yield diagnostic information.

The atrial pressure pulse

Abnormalities in the jugular pulse contour due to tricuspid disease (Fig. 2.3, p. 25) are naturally seen in the right atrial pulse as well, and analogous changes due to mitral disease are found in the *left* atrial pulse.

The arterial pressure pulse (Fig. 2.1, p. 21).

This consists of three waves—the Percussion wave (P),

separated by a shallow depression from the Tidal wave (T) and the Dicrotic wave (D) which follows the dicrotic notch marking aortic valve closure. Normally the *upstroke-time* measured from the beginning of the upstroke to the peak of pressure ranges between 0.12 and 0.16 seconds. It is shortened in conditions in which there is an aortic leak, for example aortic reflux, or patent ductus arteriosus, and prolonged if there is a fixed obstruction to outflow from the ventricle, as in aortic stenosis, when the upstroke time may range from 0.18 to 0.24 secs. In combined aortic stenosis and reflux there may be a slow upstroke with a pronounced dip between the P and the T waves resulting in the *pulsus bisferiens*. If the obstruction to left ventricular outflow is due to muscular thickening, as in obstructive cardiomyopathy, the upstroke is rapid but of small amplitude and the pressure falls to a trough between the P and T waves because the obstructing muscle contracts and restricts further outflow (Fig. 2.1, p. 21).

Shunts

In certain forms of congenital heart disease a defect in the atrial or ventricular septa or patency of the ductus arteriosus may allow abnormal passage of blood between the systemic and pulmonary circulations. As the left-sided pressures are normally higher than those on the right, the direction of flow is from left to right unless there are complicating factors. Highly oxygenated blood therefore enters the right-sided chambers and is readily detectable by sampling through a cardiac catheter. The site of the shunt can be determined by noting the point at which arterialized blood is first encountered and the amount of the shunt can be calculated by application of the Fick formula. For the pulmonary blood flow, the denominator of the Fick formula is the arterio-venous difference across the *pulmonary* capillaries; this is the arterial oxygen saturation minus the venous saturation obtained from a point distal to the shunt.

For the systemic flow the denominator is the arterio-venous difference across the systemic capillaries.

The numerator of the formula is the same in both calculations, for the quantity of oxygen taken up in the lungs can be assumed to equal that removed from the systemic capillaries.

The difference between the pulmonary and systemic flows is the amount shunted through the defect. However, the clinical significance of a shunt can be assessed simply from the ratio between the pulmonary and systemic blood flows. A moderate left to right shunt gives a ratio of 2 to 1 and larger shunts exceed this figure. If the flow ratio is less than 1.5 to 1 the shunt is not haemodynamically significant.

Techniques

Right heart catheterization

The catheter, introduced through the median cubital vein in adults and the internal saphenous vein at the groin in young children, is advanced through the right heart chambers and into the pulmonary artery and branches. It is often possible to negotiate an atrial septal defect or foramen ovale and to enter the left atrium. In Fallot's tetralogy, the aorta may be entered as well as the pulmonary artery, from the right ventricle. If the ductus arteriosus is patent the catheter can sometimes be passed through it into the aorta.

The procedure is performed under light sedation and the mortality in expert hands is probably less than 0.2 per cent of all cases. If patients with enormous cardiac enlargement are excluded, the mortality is much less.

Percutaneous left ventricular puncture

A fine gauge needle not exceeding 0.8 mm in external diameter is introduced through the position of the apex beat under local anaesthesia and light sedation. The left ventricular pressure pulse is recorded simultaneously with the brachial pulse to obtain the pressure gradient across the aortic valve, and simultaneously with the left atrial pulse as described below to obtain the gradient across the mitral valve.

Suprasternal puncture of the aorta, pulmonary artery & left atrium

Under light sedation a special needle connected to an electro-manometer is passed through the suprasternal notch at an angle of 25° to the horizontal. The position of the needle is recognized by the configuration of the pressure pulses which are monitored on an oscilloscope. A pressure record and blood sample can be obtained from the pulmonary artery in about 80 per cent of cases and from the left atrium in 99 per cent of cases. If the procedure is combined with percutaneous left ventricular puncture, the pressure gradient across the mitral valve can be accurately measured; the cardiac output is measured at the same time using the oxygen saturation of a pulmonary artery blood sample so that the degree of mitral valve obstruction can be assessed and the pulmonary vascular resistance calculated.

The safety of the procedure depends upon the dimensions of the needle which is 18.5 cm long but only 0.8 mm in external diameter. Several thousand punctures have been performed at one centre without mortality and with only infrequent and trivial complications.

Left heart catheterization by the retrograde arterial route

This is performed either by retrograde catheterization via brachial arteriotomy or by percutaneous catheterization of the femoral artery by the Seldinger technique. In the latter method a guide wire is passed through a needle introduced into the femoral artery and the needle is then withdrawn. A special catheter is then passed over the guide wire into the artery; both are then advanced a considerable distance into the aorta. The guide wire is then withdrawn and the blood in the catheter replaced with saline. The catheter is then advanced and passed retrogradely through the aortic valve into the left ventricle. If the right heart is catheterized at the same time, a blood sample is taken from the pulmonary artery for estimation of the cardiac output. If the right heart catheter is wedged in a small pulmonary artery branch so as to occlude it, the catheter transmits pressures from the pulmonary veins and left atrium (pulmonary artery wedge pressure). This pressure, recorded simultaneously with the left ventricular pressure, allows estimation of the gradient across the mitral valve. If a continuous record is made during withdrawal of the catheter from the left ventricle to the aorta, the gradient across that valve can be measured.

Left heart catheterization by the trans-septal route

In this method a catheter is passed from the internal saphenous vein at the groin to the right atrium, and a sepecial needle, introduced through it, is made to perforate the atrial septum. The catheter can then be passed over the needle into the left atrium. The needle is withdrawn and the catheter can frequently be passed into the left ventricle and withdrawn to obtain the gradient across the mitral valve. It is then withdrawn to the right atrium and right heart catheterization can then be carried out. This method is particularly useful in patients with aortic valve disease, in whom it is often difficult to pass a catheter retrogradely from the aorta into the left ventricle. It has the advantage that both sides of the heart can be catheterized from a single vessel, but it probably carries a rather higher risk (especially if left ventricular angiography is performed) than combined venous and retrograde arterial catheterization.

FURTHER READING

Mendel, D. (1974) A Practice of Cardiac Catheterization. Oxford: Blackwell Scientific Publications. 2nd edn.

4. Radiology

For appraisal of the heart size and shape it is essential that films are taken with a tube-to-patient distance of six metres. Films taken at shorter distance cause distortion of the heart outline and are valueless. This usually applies to films taken with portable X-ray apparatus in the wards. In addition to postero-anterior films two oblique views are valuable. The right anterior oblique view is taken with the patient rotated through 45° bringing the right shoulder forward to the screen or film. The left anterior oblique is taken in a similar way with the left shoulder brought forward 50 to 60°. A barium swallow is valuable in delineating the size of the left atrium especially in the right oblique view which shows the maximum backward enlargement. The contours of the heart in these projections are shown in Figure 4.1. There is now a tendency to substitute a lateral view for the oblique projections but in the author's opinion this is inferior to the oblique projections if the degree of rotation is assessed by skilled radioscopy.

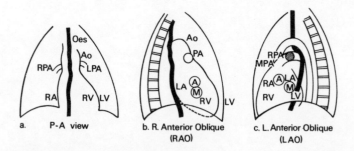

Fig. 4.1 Diagram of normal radiological appearances. Ao—Aorta; PA—Pulmonary Artery; RPA and LPA—right and left pulmonary arteries; LA—Left atrium; RA—Right atrium; RV—Right ventricle; LV—Left ventricle. A—Position of aortic valve. M—Position of mitral valve.

Although various measurements have been proposed to establish a numerical value for heart size, none has proved satisfactory and in practice a judgement based on the apearance of the heart in the three projections described is the most satisfactory method. Sometimes it is important to determine whether there has been a change in the heart size over a period of time. It is then essential to ensure that the two films under comparison are taken at a comparable phase of respiration. The films should be superimposed on a viewing box so that the first ribs coincide. If the levels of the diaphragm then coincide the cardiac outlines may be directly compared. If however the diaphragms are higher in one film the heart outline will appear larger and conversely if the diaphragm is lower the heart will appear smaller. Allowance must therefore be made for this and for about 1 cm difference between the systolic and diastolic heart size.

The radiological appearance of the lung fields is of great importance in the recognition of pulmonary oedema. This may be due to a raised left atrial pressure in mitral stenosis or left ventricular failure. Typically pulmonary oedema reproduces shadows of 'ground-glass' appearance radiating from both hilar regions. Sometimes however, the distribution of the shadows is unilateral or asymmetrical, and then confusion with pneumonia, pulmonary infarction or neoplasm may occur.

The appearance of the pulmonary arteries may suggest a high pulmonary vascular resistance if only the main branches are enlarged, and a left-to-right shunt is suggested if the smaller branches are also prominent with end-on vessels appearing as pencil-sized shadows.

In pulmonary hypertension due to mitral stenosis the arteries to the lower lobes are especially constricted and consequently the venous return from the lower zones is diminished while the veins draining the upper lobes are prominent.

Right atrial enlargement

In the P.A. view the right atrial contour exceeds 80 mm from the midline and is abnormally convex. In the left oblique view it bulges anteriorly and progressively fills in the normal retrosternal translucency. In this view, however, the right atrium is superimposed on the right ventricle and enlargement of the two chambers cannot be differentiated with certainty (Fig. 4.2)

Right ventricular enlargement

Normally the right ventricle does not reach the cardiac contour in the P.A. view and the signs of enlargement are therefore indirect, consisting of displacement of the left ventricular border to the left. However, when enlargement is great, rotation of the heart occurs so that the left ventricle is abnormally posterior; the right ventricle may then reach the left border which becomes unduly round and may be tilted upward. This is especially common in Fallot's tetralogy producing the characteristic coeur en sabot (Fig. 4.2c). In the left oblique view an enlargement of the right ventricle progressively fills the retrosternal translucency as previously described (Fig. 4.2).

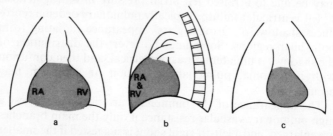

Fig. 4.2 Enlargement of the right heart. (a) The right atrium extends abnormally to the right and the cardiophrenic angle is usually obtuse. The right ventricle *may* appear on the left contour making it unduly convex. (b) In the lateral view the right atrium and ventricle are superimposed and fill the normal retro-sternal translucency. (c) Upward tilting of the apex in right ventricular hypertrophy due to Tetralogy of Fallot (Coeur en sabot)

Left atrial enlargement

The left atrium lies entirely posteriorly and is not normally seen on the cardiac contours in the P.A. view. Enlargement of the left atrial appendage however produces a convexity between the pulmonary artery and the top of the left ventricular arc. Enlargement of the right border of the left atrium may be seen as a zone of increased density within the shadow of the right atrium (Fig. 4.3a and b) but enlargement is best shown by means of a barium swallow in the right oblique position when an abrupt backward curve may be seen below the impression produced by the pulmonary artery (Fig. 4.3c).

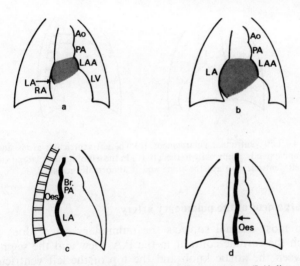

Fig. 4.3 Enlargement of the left atrium. (a) The left atrium (LA) lies at the back of the heart and does not normally appear on the cardiac contour in the PA view. If it is enlarged as in mitral stenosis, the left atrial appendage (LAA) appears as a third arc between the second arc of the pulmonary artery PA (which is usually also enlarged) and the left ventricle. Its right border may be visible within the heart shadow (LA). (b) The right border of the left atrium appears as an arc within the border of the right atrium (RA). If the left atrium is enormously enlarged its' right border may extend as low as the diaphragm with which it forms an *acute* angle. (This contrasts with the obtuse or right-angle formed by an enlarged *right* atrium with the diaphragm. (c) Right oblique view showing an enlarged left atrium displacing the barium-filled oesophagus abruptly backward immediately below the impression formed by the left bronchus (Br) and pulmonary artery (PA). (d) The PA view shows the oesophagus is displaced to the right.

Left ventricular enlargement

If hypertrophy is concentric there may be no alteration in

the cardiac outline, but if it is extreme the ventricular contour is rounded and projects unduly to the left; in the oblique position it is seen to overlap the spine. If there is dilatation as well as hypertrophy, the left ventricle is elongated downwards and to the left in the P.A. view (Fig. 4.4) as well as overlapping the spine in the left oblique view.

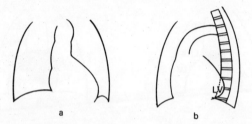

Fig. 4.4 Left ventricular enlargement. (a) The left ventricular arc is unduly long and extends abnormally to the left. (b) In the left oblique or lateral views, the left ventricle overlaps the spine and is abnormally rounded.

Enlargement of the pulmonary artery

In most normal subjects the pulmonary artery does not reach the cardiac contour in the P.A. view and the segment between the aortic knob and the top of the left ventricular curve is either straight or gently concave. However, in subjects of asthenic habitus, the heart is vertical and rotated in a clockwise direction; the pulmonary artery then appears in that segment as a gentle convexity. This must be distinguished from enlargement of the pulmonary artery which usually produces a more marked convexity (Fig. 4.3b).

Enlargement of the aorta

Post-stenotic dilatation of the ascending aorta just above the aortic valve may be recognized as a dense shadow within the contour of the right atrium (Fig. 4.5a). General enlargement of the ascending aorta may cause an abnormal convexity to the right, and unfolding of the aorta due to old age, loss of elasticity and atheroma may cause abnormal prominence of the aortic knob (Fig. 4.5b). Saccular aneurysms appear as rounded shadows which are continuous in all views with the aorta. Differentiation of shadows due to cysts, enlargement of the thyroid, and tumours of the thymus, bronchus, oesophagus or nerves may require aortography. Fusiform aneurysm of the aorta is best recognised in the left oblique view in which loss of parallelism of the aortic walls may be seen.

Calcification in the aortic knob is usually due to atheroma but in the ascending aorta it usually means syphilis.

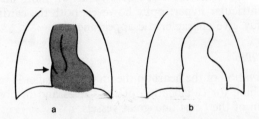

Fig. 4.5 (a) Post-stenotic dilation of the aorta in aortic valve disease is seen within the contour of the right atrium. (b) Unfolding of the aorta in atherosclerosis.

Pericardial effusion may straighten the cardiac contours so that the heart shadow becomes pear-shaped and the right cardio-phrenic angle is usually acute (Fig. 4.6). However, these appearances are by no means invariable and an effusion can produce a shadow of almost any shape.

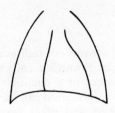

Fig. 4.6 The heart shadow in pericardial effusion. The normal contours may be straightened so that the heart appears pear-shaped. The right cardio-phrenic angle is acute.

The Accuracy of the method

In assessing concentric left ventricular hypertrophy, as in aortic stenosis or in the earlier stages of hypertension, radiology is inferior to the cardiogram. When however, there is dilatation as well as hypertrophy, as in aortic or mitral incompetence, the abnormalities are equally well shown by both methods. The slighter grades of right ventricular hypertrophy are difficult to detect by either method and bedside palpation of the heart is the most sensitive guide. In more advanced right ventricular hypertrophy however, both the cardiogram and X-ray give characteristic appearances.

Radioscopy

Observation of the heart on the image intensifier is valuable in searching for calcification of the valves and in observing pulsation of the heart and great vessels.

Calcification of the mitral and aortic valves produces shadows in characteristic positions (Figs. 4.1b and c) and they are readily distinguished from other intra-thoracic shadows by their typical elliptical movement with each heart beat.

A study of cardiac pulsations by radioscopy may be of considerable value in distinguishing enlargement of the heart shadow due to pericardial effusion from that due to intrinsic cardiac enlargement. In the former pulsations may be absent, while in the latter they may be of fairly good amplitude although it must be remembered that the greater degree of intrinsic cardiac enlargement the smaller the amplitude of pulsation.

Angiography

If a concentrated solution of radio-opaque fluid is injected rapidly into the heart through a catheter and serial pictures are taken at high speed or a cine-film made with an image intensifier, detailed information can be gained of the internal anatomy of the heart and great vessels. This has proved particularly valuable in the study of *cyanotic* congenital heart disease because the presence of a right to left shunt allows the contrast medium to delineate both sides of the heart simultaneously as well as the site and anatomy of the communication. The position and course of the great vessels can also be clearly seen. In *acyanotic* congenital heart disease, right heart angiography is not helpful because an injection of contrast medium does not usually reverse the shunt. Injection into the right heart is however valuable in differentiating pulmonary valve stenosis from infundibular stenosis and in the diagnosis of right atrial tumours and pericardial effusion.

Left ventricular angiography and aortography

This can be peformed either by the trans-septal route (p. 52) or by retrograde arterial catheterisation (p. 52). An injection of contrast medium permits visualisation of the left ventricular cavity and will demonstrate a ventricular septal defect. It allows assessement of the function of the mitral valve, demonstrating the presence and degree of mitral reflux and the mobility of the mitral cusps. Deformities due to obstructive cardiomyopathy can also be shown. An injection into the aortic root allows assessment of aortic reflux and also the demonstration of aortic aneurysms and abnormalities of the aortic arch such as coarctation.

Coronary angiography

Specially pre-formed catheters are used either percutaneously or by arteriotomy to enter the orifices of the right and left coronary arteries in turn. An injection of small amounts of contrast medium are made in several projections with high-speed cine-films of the X-ray image intensifier. Good visualisation of the main branches and their major sub-divisions can usually be obtained and serious narrowings or obstructions can be identified allowing the surgeon to plan by-pass operations in cases of angina resisting medical treatment. The procedure is not without risk but in expert hands at centres where large numbers of these investigations have been undertaken, many thousands have been performed with very low mortality.

Risks

In general, angiography slightly increases the mortality associated with catheterisation confined to pressure measurements and blood sampling: this is especially true if an intraventricular injection is made. The risk is considerably higher in infants with cyanotic congenital heart disease, but is usually acceptable as angiography may make successful surgical treatment possible.

Retrograde arterial catheterisation also involves some morbidity due to arterial thrombosis or emboli and should only be undertaken after careful consideration of the practical value of the information likely to be obtained.

FURTHER READING ..

Jefferson, K. & Rees, S. (1975) *Clinical Cardiac Radiology*. London: Butterworths.

5. Echocardiography

If a transducer capable of transmitting and receiving high frequency sound waves above the threshold of audibility (ultra sound) is placed on the chest wall and directed towards the heart, some of the waves are reflected back from the various structures lying in their path and can be detected as echoes by the transducer and converted to electronic impulses which can be recorded in the same way as an electrocardiogram. The reflecting structures include the chest wall, the pericardium if it is thickened, the right ventricular wall, the interventricular septum, the mitral valve, the left ventricular wall and sometimes the left atrium and posterior mediastinum (Fig. 5.1). Since the heart structures move with each cardiac cycle, the echoes vary correspondingly and a continuous record of them represents these movements quite accurately. They are timed using the electrocardiogram as reference

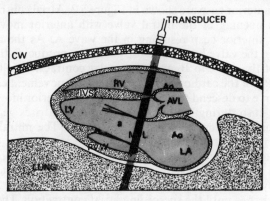

Fig. 5.1 The beam of ultra-sound traverses the right ventricular wall and cavity (RV) the intra-ventricular septum (IVS) the left ventricle (LV) the mitral valve leaflets (MVL) and the posterior ventricular wall (PVW). If the transducer is angled appropriately the beam can be made to traverse the aortic walls (AO) the aortic valve leaflets (AVL) the left atrium (LA).

tracing. Naturally the configuration of the record obtained is critically dependent on the position of the transducer on the chest and the direction of the transmitted ultra-sound beam. If the structure is not perpendicular to the beam the reflected echo may miss the transducer and fail to be recorded. The quality and nature of the record is also dependent on the acoustic properties of the structures encountered. Some reflect a high proportion of the ultra-sound waves and others, such as the lung with its contained air, reflect very little. Considerable experience is needed in positioning and directing the transducer and in interpreting the resulting records.

Echocardiography has been found to be useful in the diagnosis and evaluation of a variety of conditions and the findings in some of them are outlined here.

The movements of the mitral valve in health and disease have been extensively studied. The anterior cusp of the mitral valve moves anteriorly to open and posteriorly to close and since the cusps must obviously separate in opening and approximate in closing, the movements of the posterior cusp are the reverse of these. The echocardiogram is arranged to record an anterior movement by an upward deflection and a posterior movement by a downstroke. Normal movements of the anterior cusp are shown in Figure 5.2. Atrial contraction causes opening of the mitral valve with anterior movement of the anterior cusp resulting in the wave A. As the atrium relaxes, the valve begins to close passively, producing the descent of the curve to B, and ventricular contraction following the QRS of the cardiogram accelerates this movement causing the curve to descend to C. There is a slight anterior movement of the cusp during systole so that the tracing rises gently to the point D after the second heart sound. The mitral valve then opens abruptly with a rapid anterior motion of the anterior cusp producing a sharp upstroke to the point E. Rapid filling of the ventricle then causes the cusps to float quickly together with descent of the curve to F. There is then little change until the succeeding atrial contraction. The slope EF which represents passive closure of the mitral valve is dependent on the speed of filling of the ventricle. If this is slowed by narrowing of the mitral valve in mitral stenosis the normal slope of 50–150 mm/second is reduced in mild cases to 25–35 mm/second, in moderate cases to 15–25 mm/second, and in severe cases to less than 15 mm/second (Fig. 5.3). Mitral stenosis is, of course, not the only condition which slows ventricular filling. This occurs in all conditions with a low cardiac output and also if slowing is produced by decreased compliance of the ventricle. Mitral stenosis, however, is distinguished by an abnormal movement of the posterior cusp in addition to the decreased EF slope. Normally the posterior cusp moves in opposite directions to the anterior cusp so that the curve it produces in the echocardiogram is the mirror image of that produced by the anterior cusp,

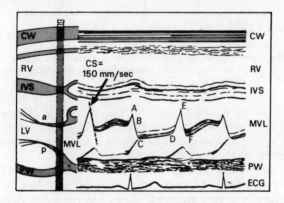

Fig. 5.2 This shows the movements of the normal mitral valve leaflets (MVL). The anterior leaflets (a) produces a characteristic M-shaped pattern for each cardiac cycle in which there are two sharp anterior movements and two sharp posterior movements producing upward and downward deflections respectively. The upward deflection occurring early in diastole (the 1st and 3rd in the diagram) is due to rapid opening of the mitral valve followed by passive closure producing a downstroke as the mitral valve floats posteriorly on the rising tide of blood in the ventricle. The second anterior deflection is due to re-opening of the valve by atrial contraction following the P wave and the second posterior deflection is due to active closure of the valve by ventricular contraction and is seen to follow the QRS wave. The posterior cusp movements are similar but opposite in direction and are only incompletely shown. However the anterior movement due to passive closure in early diastole can be seen as well as the active closure in pre-systole after which the cusps approximate to form a single line when they are closed during ventricular systole. The rate of passive closure depends upon the rate of ventricular filling. It can be measured from the closing slope (CS) and in normal subjects is between 75 and 150 mm/sec.

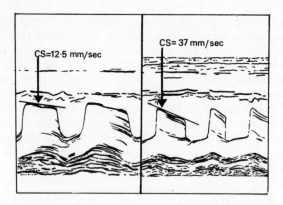

Fig. 5.3 On the left the slow closing movement of the anterior cusp of the mitral velve in mitral stenosis is seen with a closing slope of 12.5 mm/sec. Following commissurotomy passive closure is more rapid with a closing slope (CS) of 37 mm/sec. It still however does not fall within the normal range of 75 to 150 mm/sec.

though lower in amplitude. Normal motion is retained in the other conditions causing reduction of the EF slope but is lost in mitral stenosis in which there is an abnormal anterior movement of the posterior cusp in diastole.

In mitral reflux the findings are in sharp contrast with those of mitral stenosis. There is rapid filling in early diastole and consequently a very steep EF slope, but the curve does not differ greatly from normal.

In cases of prolapse of the posterior cusp of the mitral valve, there is an abnormal posterior movement of the cusp in late systole and the echoes show that the cusps are separated both in late systole and in diastole (Fig. 5.4). In hypertrophic cardiomyopathy a characteristic abnormality of movement of the mitral valve may be seen. There is an abrupt anterior movement during systole possibly owing to abnormal contraction of the anterior papillary muscle and this may contribute to the obstruction to outflow.

Echocardiography is rather less helpful in detecting abnormalities of the aortic valve than in mitral valve disease but nevertheless alterations in the rate and amplitude of opening and closure of the valve can sometimes be demonstrated. The normal echoes from the aortic valve are shown in Figure 5.5.

The method is valuable in the detection of pericardial effusion which produces an echo-free zone either anteriorly

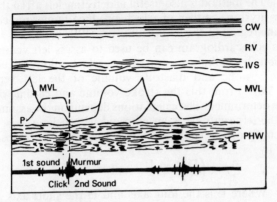

Fig. 5.4 The appearances produced by prolapse of the mitral valve leaflets due to abnormality of the chordae or voluminous cusps. The movements of the leaflets are exessive; the anterior leaflets move too far posteriorly and the posterior leaflets too far anteriorly in systole. The echoes therefore cross and do not produce a single line of a closed valve in systole. Moreover there is a characteristic posterior movement of both cusps in the latter half of systole corresponding in time to the systolic click. Following this the valve remains open and there is a systolic murmur due to reflux.

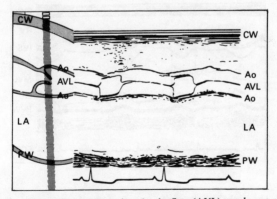

Fig. 5.5 The echoes from the aortic valve leaflets (AVL) can be seen within those from the aortic walls (AO). They can be seen to open forming a box-shaped contour during ventricular systole and come together as a single line during diastole.

between the chest wall and the right ventricle or posteriorly between the left ventricle and the mediastinum (Fig. 17. 1, p. 247). The method is also useful in detecting left atrial thrombus or myxoma, either of which produce numerous echoes from the region of the left atrium (Fig. 19.1, p. 253).

The echocardiogram can be used to assess left ventricular function, by making measurements which allow calculation of the systolic and diastolic volume of the left ventricle (Fig. 5.6). From this the stroke volume and cardiac output can be determined. The calculations depend on the assumption that the left ventricle is an ellipsoid with a long axis, twice the length of the short axis. The volume of an ellipsoid is given by:

$$V = \frac{4}{3}\pi \times \left(\frac{D}{2}\right)^2 \times \frac{L}{2}$$

Where L is the long axis and D the short axis
If L = 2D

$$V = \frac{4}{3}\pi \times \frac{D^3}{4}$$

Since π is approxiately 3
$V = D^3$ approx.

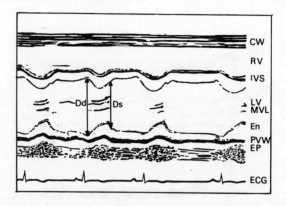

Fig. 5.6 The stroke volume can be estimated by subtracting the cube of the minimum dimension in systole (Ds) from the cube of the maximum dimension in diastole (Ds) at the peak of the R waves. En-Endocardium, other symbols as in Fig. 5.1.

FURTHER READING

Feigenbaum, H. (1977) *Echocardiography*. 2nd edn. Philadelphia: Lea and Fibiger.

6. Electrocardiography

Introduction and definitions

The electrocardiogram is a graphic record of the electrical changes which produce myocardial contraction. These changes consist of the successive depolarisation and repolarisation of the cells. Heart muscle cells and those of the specialised sino-atrial and atrio-ventricular nodes are bounded by cell membranes which are relatively permeable to potassium and impermeable to sodium ions. An enzyme system, the sodium pump, tends to transfer sodium ions out of the cell and potassium ions into it. Intracellular potassium is high and sodium low while the reverse is true of extracellular fluid. Potassium tends to leak from this high intracellular concentration, but leaves behind it corresponding anions to which the membrane is not permeable. This flow of potassium down the concentration gradient continues until it is balanced by the unopposed negativity of the anions within. When this equilibrium is reached there is a potential difference across the membrane of –90 mV and this is called the resting potential (Fig. 6.1). The cell is then in a polarised state and resembles a charged capacitor. When depolarisation occurs the cell membrane abruptly becomes permeable to sodium and calcium ions which enter abolishing the transmembrane potential difference and even causing temporary intracellular positivity. This limits the further entry of sodium. These electrical changes stimulate adjacent cells to undergo similar depolarisation and the process spreads throughout the heart muscle. This however takes time and it follows that some portions are depolarised while others are still polarised and a potential difference exists between them. This creates an electrical field which can be detected by electrodes on the surface of the body and can be recorded by the electrocardiograph. Since depolarised cells are electrically negative with

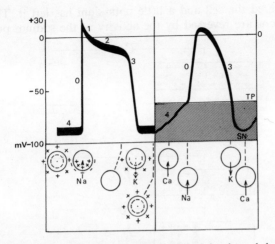

Fig. 6.1 Transmembrane action potentials. The left-hand panel shows transmembrane action potentials from the myocardial cell and the right-hand
panel those from a cell from the sino-atrial node. The ionic changes in the
cells are shown diagramatically beaneath each panel. Phase 4 is the resting
polarised state and myocardial cells carry a positive surface charge due to
slow leakage of potassium. Intra-cellular potential is about -90 mV. With
depolarisation (phase zero) there is a rapid influx of sodium causing
temporary inter-cellular positivity (phase one). There is then a plateau (phase
two) until influx of calcium and then the leakage of potassium causes repolarisation during phase three until the resting polarised state is regained.
The right-hand panel shows specialised sino-atrial cells undergoing a slow
spontaneous depolarisation through influx of calcium in phase four. This
occurs until a threshold potential is reached at about -70 mV when abrupt
depolarisation through influx of sodium occurs. Repolarisation (phase three)
begins almost at once, without an intervening plateau, due to gradual leakage
of potassium. (TP–Threshold Potential, SN–Sinus Node).

respect to polarised cells it follows that an advancing wave
front of activation carries before it a zone of positive electrical
potential and a retreating wave front a negative potential
(Fig. 6.2). The direction successively followed from moment
to moment by these wave fronts therefore determines the
size and direction of the deflections of the electrocardiogram.

Repolarisation occurs through loss of the membrane permeability to sodium and a gradual leakage of potassium
previously described which produces surface positivity. As a
result of the electrical cycle it will be noted that a little sodium

has entered the cell and a little potassium has left it. These alterations are reversed by the activity of the sodium pump

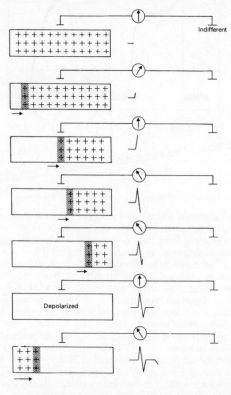

Fig. 6.2 Electrocardiography. The rectangle represents a muscle strip carrying surface positive charges in the resting polarised state. The second rectangle shows depolarisation beginning at the left-hand end with the abolition of surface positively. This means that the adjacent polarised cells are positive with respect to the depolarised cells and an advancing wave front (shaded) of positivity approaches the electrode giving an upstroke in the recorded electro-cardiogram. The upstroke increases in height until the wave of positivity reaches the electrode when it abruptly reverses and becomes negative as the wave front retreats from the electrode. Maximum negativity occurs just as the wave-front passes the electrode and negativity diminishes as it becomes more distant. When the whole muscle strip is depolarised the deflection returns to the base-line. As repolarisation begins at the left-hand end of the muscle strip a wave-front of *negativity* approaches the electrode giving a downstroke which reverses as it passes beneath the electrode.

previously mentioned, which probably acts throughout systole and diastole.

The electrical activity of the cell during depolarisation and repolarisation just described is called the trans-membrane action potential and its time course is represented in Figure 6.1. Two types of action potential are shown: that on the left represents the action potential of a myocardial cell and that on the right the action potential from the sino-atrial node. Important differences exist between them. The arrival of an impulse at a myocardial cell produces rapid depolarisation followed by a plateau and then rapid repolarisation (phase 3) with return to the resting potential which remains unchanged as the flat phase 4 throughout diastole. By contrast the sino-atrial node undergoes slow spontaneous depolarisation during diastole and phase 4 is consequently inclined and not flat. This slow spontaneous diastolic depolarisation is probably mediated by the entry of calcium into the cell rather than sodium. When the entry of these postive ions causes the intracellular potential to reach about $-75mV$ a threshold is reached at which the membrane becomes abruptly permeable to sodium causing rapid depolarisation (phase 0). This is followed almost immediately without an intervening plateau by rapid repolarisation (phase 3). This spontaneous depolarisation or automaticity produces regular impulses which cause depolarisation of the myocardial fibres. This property is also possessed by the A–V junctional tissue and the His-Purkinje cells. The rate at which they produce impulses depends upon the rate of diastolic depolarisation shown diagrammatically by the slope of phase 4. If this is steep as in the sino-atrial node the threshold potential is reached quickly and impulses are discharged frequently. Diastolic depolarisation occurs more slowly in A–V junctional tissue and still more slowly in His-Purkinje cells (Fig. 6.3). The inherent rhythmicity in adult man is about 70 to 80 per minute for the sino-atrial node, 40 to 50 per minute for the A–V junctional tissue, and 30 to 40 per minute for the His-Purkinje cells. These three specialised tissues are potential pacemakers and it can be seen that the fastest one, the sino-atrial node, will discharge the two slower ones because it produces a fresh depolarising impulse before the diastolic depolarisation of the slower centres reaches

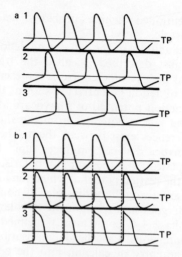

Fig. 6.3 (a) The transmembrane action potentials of: (1) The sino-atrial node (2) The AV node and, (3) The His-Purkinje cells. Spontaneous diastolic depolarisation occurs fastest, (producing the steepest upstroke) in the sino-atrial node and slowest (with the flattest upstroke) in the His-Purkinje cells. Discharge is therefore fastest in the sino atrial node, slower in the AV node and slowest in the His-Purkinje cells. The lower half of the diagram (b) shows that the faster discharging rate of the SA node discharges both the lower two nodes before they reach threshold potential (TP). The AV node can only become effective if the sino-atrial node is inoperative and the His-Purkinje cells are only effective if both the upper two nodes are inoperative.

threshold. If the sino-atrial node is not working, the A–V junctional node will operate and discharge the His-Purkinje cells, which will only become operative if both the upper two pacemakers are inoperative.

Following phase 0 there is an absolute refractory period during which a further stimulus will not produce a response. Then after phase 3 has begun, there is a relative refractory period lasting until the beginning of phase 4 during which a stronger than normal stimulus will produce a response (Fig. 6.4). The relative refractory period corresponds to the T wave of the cardiogram, when the muscle cells have reached varying degrees of repolarization. This accounts for the vulnerability of the myocardium at this time when a premature beat can induce ventricular fibrillation.

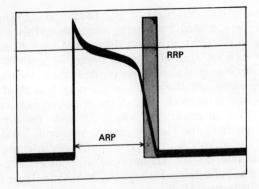

Fig. 6.4 The action potential of a myocardial cell. The cell is absolutely refractory to a further stimulus from the time of depolarisation until after repolarisation has begun (ARP). It is then relatively refractory, requiring a stronger than normal stimulus to produce a response, until repolarisation is complete (RRP). The period corresponds with the T wave of the cardiogram when the myocardial cells have reached varying degrees of repolarisation. This lack of uniform responsiveness leads to the possibility of ventricular fibrillation in response to a premature beat at this period.

The genesis of the electrocardiographic deflections

The potential changes produced by depolarisation in the sino-atrial node are too small to be recorded from the body surface, but the spread of depolarisation across the atria produces an electrical field which can be so recorded. Depolarisation of the atria produces a blunt upright deflection called the P wave. When the impulse reaches the A–V node a physiological delay occurs allowing time for complete filling of the ventricle. During this interval repolarisation of the atria begins and it is completed during and after the spread of the impulse through the ventricles described below. The potential changes due to repolarisation produce a field equal in magnitude but opposite in direction to those of depolarisation and so cause a shallow negative wave, the atrial T wave (Ta) on which is superimposed the QRS wave due to depolarisation of the ventricles.

The electrical changes produced by depolarisation of the A–V node, bundle of His, bundle branches and Purkinje network (the His-Purkinje system) are too small to produce a detectable electrical field at the body surface. They can however be recorded by placing electrode catheters transvenously in the right atrium. A diagram of such a recording together with a surface electrocardiogram is shown in Figure 6.5. The beginning of the P wave of the surface electrocardiogram represents depolarisation in the neighbourhood of the SA node and is scarecely seen in the His bundle electrogram (HBE). After an interval of about 30 msec. the arrival of depolarisation in the vicinity of the A–V node produces a series of deflections A in the His bundle electrogram. There follows an interval (the AH interval) of about 90 msec during which the impulse passes through the A–V node. There follows a sharp deflection H due to passage through the bundle of His. There is then a further interval, the H–V interval, occupied by travel of the impulse down the bundle branches and Purkinje network. Ventricular activation is marked by a series of very large amplitude rapid deflections V. The H–V interval measures about 40 msec.

Depolarisation of the ventricle spreads from the endocardial surfaces towards the epicardial surfaces by contiguity as in the atrium. There is a fairly constant sequence of depolarisation

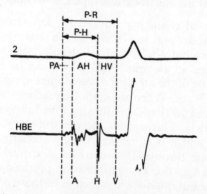

Fig. 6.5 The His bundle electrocardiogram (HBE). The P–A interval of 30 msec represents the conduction time from the region of the S–A node to a point low in the right atrium. The H deflection represents depolarization in the His bundle and the A–H interval of 90 msec represents conduction through the A–V junctional tissues. The V deflections represent the onset of depolarization of the ventricle and the H–V interval of 40 msec therefore represents the conduction time of the His-Purkinje system.

of the various parts of the ventricle and this gives the resultant QRS complex a characteristic configuration. After the QRS complex there is a short interval in which potential changes are small or absent and the galvanometer returns to the isoelectric line; this is the beginning of the S–T segment. Repolarisation of the ventricle then begins but it occurs at a slower speed and by a different path from that of depolarisation so that the T wave it produces may have the same direction as the QRS, but is broad and blunt.

Following the T wave a small blunt deflection of uncertain origin, the U wave is sometimes seen.

Nomenclature and definitions of the deflections

The following definitions of the waves of the cardiogram shown in Figures 6.6 (b) must be memorized.

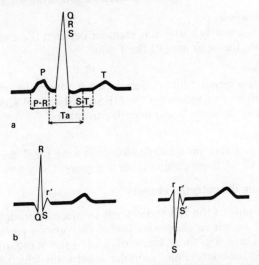

Fig. 6.6 The deflections of the electrocardiogram. (a) The P wave is a small (upto 2.5 mm) slightly notched deflection. It is upright in most leads and has a maximum duration of 0.11 sec. It may be followed by a shallow depression (Ta) produced by atrial repolarization. The QRS deflection is superimposed on the Ta wave the latter part of which coincides with the S–T segment. The interval between the P wave and the QRS complex is called the P–R interval and measures 0.12–0.21 sec depending on age and heart rate. (b) Varieties of the QRS complex. The duration of the QRS is 0.08–0.1 sec (see text).

The P wave

This is a blunt upright deflection less than 2.5 mm in amplitude and 0.11 sec duration preceding the QRS complex.

The Ta wave

This is a shallow negative deflection following the P wave and the QRS is superimposed on it.

The QRS complex

The Q wave. This is the first downward deflection which is followed by an upward one. If no upward deflection is present a downward deflection must be called QS.

The R wave is the first upward deflection.

The S wave is a downward deflection which follows an R wave.

The R' wave is an upright deflection following the S wave

The S' wave is a negative deflection following an R' wave

The ST segment

This is a nearly horizontal segment between the end of the QRS and the beginning of the T wave.

The T wave

This is a broad, blunt deflection arising from the end of the ST segment and following the QRS by about 0.4 seconds. It is positive in some leads, negative in others.

The U wave

This is a tiny broad deflection following the T wave.

Not all of these components are present in every lead.

Recording the potential changes

Each pole of the galvanometer is connected through a lead selector switch to electrodes placed on various parts of the body. There are three kinds of leads—the standard leads, unipolar limb leads, and unipolar chest leads which are also called V leads.

1. *The standard leads*

The connections are conventionally made as follows:

Lead 1 = Right arm (−) and left arm (+)
Lead 2 = Right arm (−) and left leg (+)
Lead 3 = Left arm (−) and left leg (+)

The signs in parentheses indicate the positive and negative poles of the galvanometer which is arranged to record an upstroke if the potential at the postive pole exceeds that of the negative pole. In the standard leads the galvanometer is simultaneously influenced by potential variations at each of the two electrodes and it records their algebraic sum.

The lead *axis* is a hypothetical line joining the electrode positions and indicating, in the case of the limb leads, the direction of the lead in the frontal plane. It is convenient to draw the three lead axes through the same zero point as shown in Figure 6.7.

2. *The unipolar limb leads, and augmented unipolar limb leads*

In unipolar limb leads the galvanometer is arranged to record the potential variations from only one limb at a time instead of recording the algebraic sum of two as in the standard leads. This is achieved by connecting one pole of the galvano-meter to a central terminal which is connected to all three limbs. The sum of the potential variations of these three limbs is zero, so that the terminal remains at zero potential through-out the cardiac cycle. The other pole of the galvanometer is connected in turn to each of the three limbs. Recorded in this way, however, the deflections are inconveniently small but they can be increased without altering their configuration by disconnecting the lead being explored from the central terminal.

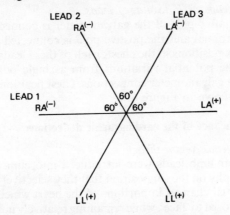

Fig. 6.7 The axes and galvanometer connections of the standard limb leads

Recorded in this way the leads are called *augmented* unipolar limb leads AVR, AVL and AVF. Their galvanometer connections and lead axes are shown in Figure 6.8.

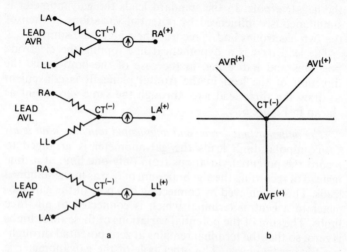

Fig. 6.8 (a) The galvanometer connections of the augmented unipolar limb leads. (b) The axes of the augmented unipolar limb leads. (CT–Central Terminal).

3. *Chest leads or V (voltage) leads*

The negative pole of the galvanometer is connected to the central terminal and the positive pole is connected in turn to each of six positions in the chest; each of these leads therefore records the potential variations from a single point on the chest. The galvanometer connections, chest positions and lead axes are shown in Figure 6.9.

The significance of the cardiographic deflections

Unipolar versus vector theory

Unipolar limb leads were introduced into clinical electrocardiography on the supposition that they selectively recorded the potential changes in portions of the heart which the leads were supposed to 'face', while remaining relatively uninfluenced by the potential changes in the remainder of the heart. This

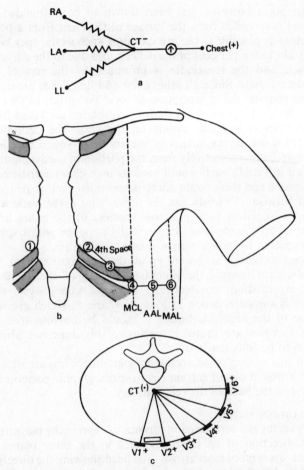

Fig. 6.9 (a) The galvanometer connection of the 'V' leads. (b) The position of the chest electrodes for leads V1–6. V1 and V2 are in the 4th inter-space immediately to the right and left of the sternum respectively. V4 is in the 5th inter-space in the mid-clavicular line (MCL) V3 is half-way between V2 and V4. V5 and V6 lie on a horizontal line projected from the V4 position to the mid-axillary line. V5 is at the point where this line intersects the anterior axillary line (AAL) and V6 is at the point where this line meets the mid-axillary line (MAL). (c) The axes of leads V1–6 are indicated in the diagram of a transverse section of the thorax viewed from above. CT denotes the central terminal.

assumption however, has been shown to be unfounded. If a lead is recorded from the surface of the chest from a point as close as possible to the myocardium, such as the apex beat, only about ten per cent of the deflection is due to the adjacent muscle and the remainder is produced by the rest of the cardiac muscle. Since all other chest and limb leads are much more remote, the contribution of local potentials to them is even less. Also it has been shown that if leads are taken from diametrically opposite points on the chest the deflections recorded are mirror images of one another. Now if each lead were recording selectively from the portion of cardiac muscle which it 'faced', each would have its own characteristic configuration and there ought not to be any mirror image relationship between the leads. On the other hand if the leads were simply recording total potential changes of the entire heart then records made from diametrically opposite points would be expected to show a mirror-image relationship.

Vector theory is based upon the assumption that the cardiogram records the potential changes of the whole of the myocardium unselectively, with the sole proviso that there is some distortion in leads V.4. and 5. which are very close to the heart. Although it should be obvious that the two theories are mutually exclusive this does not always seem to be fully realized.

In this section some vectorcardiographic terms are defined and explanations of certain electrocardiographic patterns are given on the basis of the vector theory.

The cardiac vectors

A vector is a term used in physics to express the magnitude and direction of an electrical force in the three planes of space. Its symbol is an arrow—the head showing the direction and the length indicating the magnitude of the force. A cardiac vector expresses the magnitude and direction of the sum of all the electrical forces of the heart at a given moment. Since depolarization of the whole heart does not occur instantaneously but spreads through the muscle in a complicated sequence in time and space, there are a series of different *momentary* vectors for depolarization (QRS vectors) and another series of momentary vectors for repolarization (T wave vectors). Each series can be averaged to give a *mean* QRS vector and a *mean* T wave vector. If depolarization and repolarization followed the same time sequence, the first portion of cardiac muscle to be depolarized, would be the first portion to be repolarized and the QRS and T wave vectors would be equal and opposite. In terms of the conventional scalar cardiogram, this would mean that the direction and shape of the QRS and T waves would be nearly equal and opposite in all leads. However, repolarization follows a slower and different course so that the T wave vector normally points in much the *same* direction as the QRS and is smaller and broader.

The deflections in the limb leads depend on the direction of the cardiac vector in the frontal plane and those of the chest leads depend on its direction in the horizontal plane.

In considering the genesis of cardiographic deflections two principles must be remembered:

1. The galvanometer connections are arranged so that a vector directed towards the positive pole records an upstroke, while one directed away from it gives a downstroke.

2. The magnitude of the deflection depends upon the angle between the lead axis and the vector. The maximum deflection is produced when the vector is parallel with the lead axis and zero when it is at right angles to the lead axis. This will be readily understood if the vector is represented as an arrow between a light source and the lead axis. The largest 'shadow' is cast when the arrow is parallel to the lead axis and none when it is perpendicular to it (Fig. 6.10).

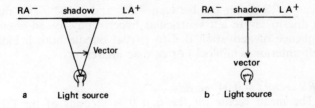

Fig. 6.10 The relation between the direction of the vector and the size of the cardiographic deflection. (a) The vector produces the largest deflection in the lead to which it is most nearly parallel. (see text). (b) It causes the smallest deflection in the lead most nearly at right angles to it.

The direction of the mean QRS vectors

The direction of the mean QRS vector in the frontal plane can be estimated quite simply by inspection of the limb lead deflections and the application of the two foregoing principles. The lead showing the largest net area under the QRS deflection is the one most parallel to the QRS vector. To obtain the net area under the QRS deflection the number of small squares above the isoelectric line is added algebraically to those enclosed below the isoelectric line. If the deflection is predominantly upright, the vector is pointing towards the positive pole of the lead, while the reverse is true if it is predominantly negative. Since the lead axes are at angles of 60° to one another the direction of the cardiac vectors can be expressed in degrees using the axis of lead 1 as a reference (Fig. 6.11). Normally the QRS vector lies between −30° and +100° and this is called the mean electrical axis. Its direction depends upon the patient's age and bodily configuration. In children, in whom the right ventricle is preponderant, the axis is nearly vertical at about +90°; in adolescence it progressively shifts to the left, its final position depending upon the bodily habitus. Tall, asthenic individuals retain a relatively vertical axis, while short, stocky individuals tend to have a more horizontal axis between zero and −30°.

Right axis deviation is said to be present if the axis of the mean QRS vector exceeds +90°. It usually indicates right ventricular hypertrophy.

Left axis deviation is said to be present if the axis of the mean QRS vector lies between −30° and −180°. This may be due to severe left ventricular hypertrophy, or an altered sequence of activation due to partial bundle branch block (left anterior hemiblock) or cardiac infarction.

QRS vectors at 0.04 seconds

The mean vector for the first 0.04 seconds of the QRS complex usually lies in the same direction as the mean vector for the whole complex. This means that if the QRS is upright, as it is in most leads, the deflection during the first 0.04 secs. of the QRS is also predominantly upright and any negative deflection (Q wave) must necessarily be small in magnitude and brief in duration. In cardiac infarction however, the direction

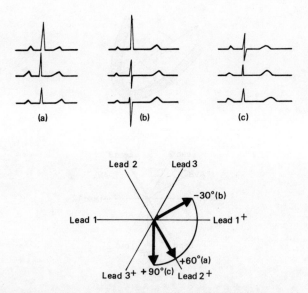

Fig. 6.11 The normal range of QRS axis and its estimation by inspection of the limb leads. In (a) the QRS of lead 2 encloses the maximum area and this is therefore the axial lead. Since it is upright the vector is directed toward its positive pole and the axis is +60°. In (b) the QRS of lead 1 encloses the maximum net area and since it is upright the general direction of the vector is toward its positive pole. Since the QRS in lead 2 is nearly equiphasic, the net area enclosed by it approaches zero and the vector must be nearly at right angles to this lead. The axis is therefore about −30°. If the S wave is dominant in lead 2 the vector would be directed toward its negative pole. The axis would lie between −30° and −90° and this would be abnormal left axis deviation. In (c) the QRS in lead 1 is equiphasic and the mean vector is therefore perpendicular to this lead. Since QRS 2 and 3 are upright there is right axis deviation of +90°. If the S is dominant in lead 1 the vector would point toward the negative pole of lead 1 and the right axis deviation exceeding +90° would be abnormal.

of the 0.04 sec vector is characteristically altered, pointing away from the infarct, and away from the mean vector which lies in the axis of the left ventricle.

The 0.04 sec vector thus points towards the negative pole of one or other of the limb leads and results in large and prolonged Q waves characteristic of cardiac infarction (Fig. 6.12).

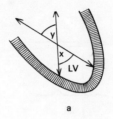

a

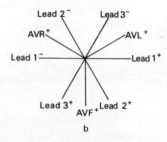

b

Fig. 6.12 (a) The direction of the initial (0.04 sec) and mean vectors in cardiac infarction. The direction of the mean QRS vector roughly corresponds to the long axis of the left ventricle and lies in the range of the angle (x). In cardiac infarction the 0.04 sec vector points in an opposite direction within the range of the angle (y). (b) It therefore points to the negative pole of the limb leads and results in deep Q waves exceeding 0.03 secs duration in one or more of these leads.

The mean T wave vector

This can be estimated in exactly the same way as the QRS vector. Usually it lies within 50° of the mean QRS vector and a value exceeding this indicates disease—usually hypertrophy or ischaemia.

Abnormalities of the P wave

Right atrial hypertrophy

The first portion of the P wave is produced by the right atrium and is separated by a slight notch from the portion produced by the left atrium. The impulse passes through the right atrium in an inferior direction roughly parallel with the axes of leads 2 or 3 and Vl. Right atrial hypertrophy therefore causes tall pointed P waves exceeding 2.5 mm in these leads (Fig. 6.13). The longer time taken for the impulse to spread through the enlarged atrium prolongs the duration of the right atrial component which then overlaps that of the left atrium so that the whole P wave is not widened.

Left atrial hypertrophy

The impulse passes laterally and backwards into the left atrium in a direction approximately parallel to Leads 1 and V.6. The changes due to left atrial hypertrophy are therefore best seen in those leads and consist of exaggeration of the notch and prolongation and slight enlargement of the second half of the P wave. The total duration of the P wave may exceed the normal maximum of 0.11 sec (Fig. 6.13)

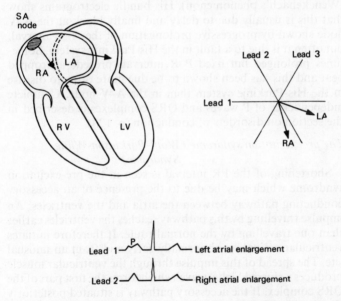

Fig. 6.13 The genesis of the P wave. The impulse spreads inferiorly from the SA node across the right atrium and its mean vector (RA) is therefore in the axis of lead 2. Right atrial hypertrophy therefore produces a tall pointed P wave in lead 2. Activation of the left atrium occurs later and proceeds laterally right-to-left so that the meant vector (LA) is in the axis of lead 1. Left atrial hypertrophy therefore produces a late peak in the P wave broadening and notching it in lead 1.

Abnormalities of the P–R interval

The P–R interval is measured from the beginning of the P wave to the beginning of the QRS (if a Q wave is present the interval measured is actually P–Q and not P–R). Normal values are about 0.08–0.12 secs. for infants, 0.10–0.16 for children and 0.12–0.21 for adults. Prolongation of the P–R interval may be caused by digitalis, rheumatic fever, ischaemic heart disease and undetermined causes. His bundle electrograms show that prolongation is usually due to delay in the A–V node with prolongation of the A–H interval. Sometimes the prolongation is phasic, the P–R interval progressively lengthening until the ventricle fails to respond. After the pause so produced the cycle begins again with a normal P–R interval (Wenckebach's phenomenon). His-bundle electrograms show that this is usually due to delay and finally block at the A–V node shown by progressive prolongation of the A–H interval, but often it is due to a fault in the His-Purkinje system. Sometimes prolonged but fixed P–R intervals precede a dropped beat and this has been shown to be due more often to disease in the His-Purkinje system than in the A–V node. Complete independence of P waves and QRS complexes is described in the section on disorders of conduction (p. 123).

The pre-excitation syndrome (Wolff-Parkinson-White Syndrome)

Shortening of the PR interval is seen in the pre-excitation syndrome which may be due to the presence of an accessory conducting pathway between the atria and the ventricles. An impulse travelling by this pathway reaches the ventricles earlier than one travelling by the normal route. It therefore initiates ventricular activation abnormally early and from an unusual site. The spread of this impulse through the ventricular muscle produces a slurred 'delta-wave' which forms the first part of the QRS complex. If the accessory pathway is situated posteriorly the abnormally early activation of the ventricle proceeds in an anterior direction giving an upwardly directed delta-wave in lead 1 and the chest leads, which it is approaching. If the accessory pathway is situated anteriorly activation proceeds in a posterior direction giving upright delta-waves in leads 2, 3 and VF. The degree of deformity of the whole QRS complex produced by the delta-wave is variable. It may be slight affecting only its early part or considerable with great broadening of the QRS. The PR interval is shortened by the delta-wave which correspondingly lengthens the duration of the QRS complex (Fig. 6.14).

The condition is of clinical significance because a reciprocating mechanism may occur. An atrial ectopic beat may find the accessory pathway refractory and descend by the normal route to activate the ventricle; it may then immediately return to the atrium by the now non-refractory accessory pathway and then descend again by the normal route, producing a circus movement of the impulse with consequent rapid ventricular stimulation resulting in paroxysm of tachycardia (p. 103).

In another variety of pre-excitation the accessory pathway by-passes the AV node or travels unduly fast through it and then rejoins the bundle of His. In these cases there is a short PR interval but since conduction to the ventricles is through the bundle of His and its branches in a normal fashion the QRS complex is not broadened. However this anomaly too may be associated with paroxysmal tachycardia as previously explained.

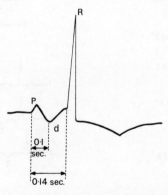

Fig. 6.14 The pre-excitation syndrome. Fast conduction through an accessory pathway leads to premature activation of the ventricle producing a delta wave (d) which shortens the P–R interval to 0.1 sec and deforms the QRS. The interval from the beginning of P to the beginning of the normal QRS is 0.14 sec.

Abnormalities of the QRS complex

Ventricular hypertrophy

Hypertrophy of either ventricle causes an increase in magnitude of the mean QRS vector and an increased tendency for it to point in the long axis of the affected ventricle. As a result changes may occur in axis deviation and in the voltage of the deflections in the limb or chest leads or both. The T vector may be altered and point in a direction opposite to that of the QRS vector. The reason for this is uncertain, but in right or left ventricular hypertrophy, the diagnosis is secure only if both QRS and S–T–T wave changes are present. QRS abnormalities alone must be interpreted with caution especially in young or thin patients. If S–T–T wave changes are present alone the differential diagnosis of such abnormalities must be considered. (see p. 94).

Left ventricular hypertrophy. There may be left axis deviation particularly in adults or elderly subjects in whom the vector

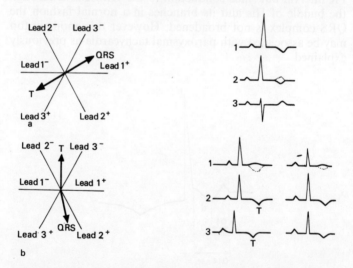

Fig. 6.15 (a) Left ventricular hypertrophy with left axis deviation. Lead 1 is the axial lead showing tall voltage. The opposite direction of the T vector produces T wave inversion in lead 1 and flattening or inversion in lead 2. (b) Left ventricular hypertrophy with normal axis. Lead 2 or 3 is the axial lead showing tall voltage and T wave inversion.

normally tends in this direction. Lead 1 is then the axial lead with an R wave exceeding 12 mm and an inverted T wave. In younger subjects however, the axis may be normal and all three limb leads show the abnormalities (Fig. 6.15 a and b).

In the chest leads the increased voltage may produce a deep S wave in V1 or 2, and a tall R wave in V6, the sum of the two exceeding 35 mm. Higher limits are set in children or thin persons. As in the limb leads the S–T–T vectors point in the opposite direction to the QRS.

The direction of the QRS vector in the frontal and horizontal planes determines the magnitude of the QRS complexes in the limb and chest leads. If it remains nearly *parallel* to the *frontal plane*, in which the limb leads and V6 lie, these will show a large deflection. If it is directed markedly posteriorly however

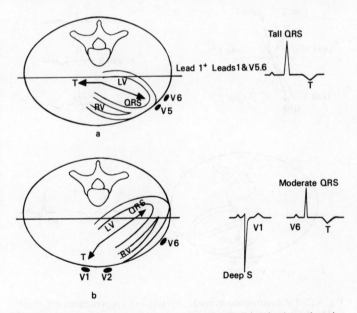

Fig. 6.16 The voltage in left ventricular hypertrophy. (a) A horizontal section of the thorax showing the long axis of the left ventricle lying approximately parallel to the frontal plane. Hypertrophy then results in large voltage R waves in lead 1 and leads V5 and V6. (b) If the long axis is directed more posteriorly it is more nearly parallel to the axes of V1 or V2 which therefore show large voltage S waves.

(as may well be the case since the left ventricle lies at the back of the heart) it is *parallel* to *leads V*1 *and* 2 and these show large voltage, while deflections in the limb leads and V6 are small (Fig. 6.16).

Right ventricular hypertrophy. The QRS vector shifts rightwards and anteriorly often producing right axis deviation particularly in children or young adults and causing lead 2 or 3 to become the axial lead with an R wave exceeding 12 mm. In addition the vector points forwards in the horizontal plane towards lead V1 which shows a dominant R wave and away from V6 which shows a dominant S wave (Fig. 6.17).

The shift of the S–T and T vectors in the opposite direction to the QRS vector causes the S–T depression and T wave inversion in the leads with the tall R waves.

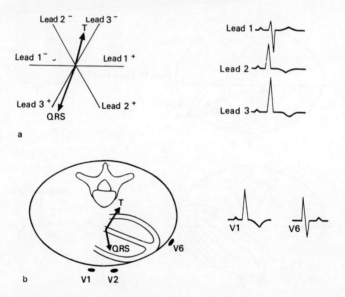

Fig. 6.17 Right ventricular hypertrophy. (a) Lead 1 is predominantly negative and lead 3 is the axial lead so that there is right axis deviation of about +120° The T vector points in the opposite direction so that the T waves may be inverted in leads 2 and 3. (b) The mean QRS vector is directed anteriorly towards V1 and perpendicular to V6 and the T vector is in the opposite direction. V1 therefore shows a dominant R wave with inverted T waves and V6 an equiphasic QRS with upright T waves.

Bundle branch block

Interruption, whether functional or organic, of the specialized conducting bundles slows the spread of the impulse through the affected ventricle and therefore prolongs the duration of the QRS complex beyond the normal limit of 0.11 sec; it also alters the sequence of activation, causing characteristic alterations of the QRS pattern. The S–T and T vectors are also abnormal and point in the opposite direction to the mean QRS vectors as in ventricular hypertrophy.

Left bundle branch block. Normally the left ventricle is activated slightly before the right and produces rightward initial vectors giving normal Q waves in lead 1 and leads V.4–6. In left branch block this sequence is reversed, for the impulse spreads from the right ventricle to the left, abolishing the Q waves and producing slurred R waves in the axial limb leads and V.4–6. The QRS duration is 0.12 secs or more. The abnormal S–T and T vectors produce S–T and T wave inversion in the leads with the tallest R waves (Fig. 6.18a).

Right bundle branch block. The late activation of the right ventricle, when excitation of the left ventricle is complete, produces a late vector directed anteriorly and to the right. Reference to Figure 6.18b shows that this produces a deep broad S wave in lead 1 and a terminal R wave in V.1. while the QRS duration is prolonged beyond the normal 0.11 sec. There are abnormal S–T and T vectors in the opposite direction and so there is S–T depression and T wave inversion in leads 2, 3 and V.1–3.

Low voltage. Abnormally low voltage of the cardiogram is said to be present if the sum of all the R and S waves in the limb leads is less than 15 mm or if the largest deflections (R + S) in the precordial leads is less than 9 mm. The amplitude of the T waves is usually proportionately reduced. The possible causes are:

1. Old age
2. Myxoedema
3. Severe anaemia (under 5 g/dl)
4. Pericarditis with effusion or constriction
5. Severe emphysema
6. Diffuse myocardial fibrosis
7. Oligaemic shock

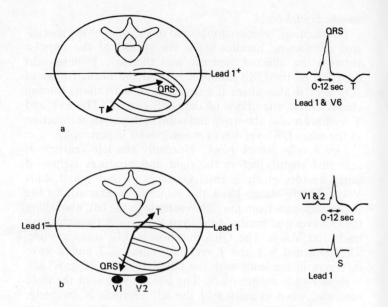

Fig. 6.18 (a) Left bundle branch block. (a) Activation of the right ventricle occurs first and spreads to the left ventricle. The QRS vector is therefore directed to the left toward lead 1+ and V6 throughout the cardiac cycle and these leads show slurred R waves and no Q waves. S–T and T vectors point in the opposite direction and there is S–T depression and T wave inversion in these leads. (b) Right bundle branch block. The *late* activation of the right ventricle produces a *late* vector directed anteriorly and to the right towards the negative pole of lead 1 and the positive pole of V1. These leads therefore show prominent S and R waves respectively

With the exception of myxoedema which characteristically shows bradycardia these conditions are usually accompanied by tachycardia.

Abnormalities of the S–T segment and T waves

Abnormal elevation or depression of the S–T segments should be sought by placing a straight edge or drawing a line from the beginning of the upstroke of one P wave to a similar point on the next P wave. The S–T segment should normally lie along this line or slightly above it, the only exception being the depression caused by the atrial T wave (q.v.). This causes depression of both the P–R interval and the S–T segment so that the two can be seen to lie on a continuous curve.

Normally the S–T segment is isoelectric or 0.5 mm elevated in leads 1, 2 and V.4–6 while it may be elevated as much as 2.0 mm in V.1–3. It is never normally depressed more than 0.5 mm. The T wave is normally upright in leads 1, 2 and V.2–6 in adults. It is normally inverted in leads V.1–3 in children and adolescents.

Acute epicardial ischaemia

The injured muscle surrounding the necrotic centre of an infarct gives rise to a current of injury which produces S–T elevation. The T wave is at first flattened and may be invisible but later, inversion occurs before the S–T segment returns to normal (Fig. 6.19a). If S–T elevation is present in leads 1 and V.6. due to an anterior injury there is *reciprocal* depression in lead 3, and if the S–T elevation is present in lead 3 due to a posterior injury there is reciprocal depression in lead 1 and V.2–5.

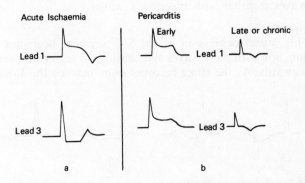

Fig. 6.19 S–T elevation. (a) Acute epicardial ischaemia. S–T elevation in one lead is accompanied by reciprocal depression in another. The T wave begins to invert before the S–T elevation returns to the baseline. (b) Acute pericarditis. S–T elevation is present in several leads without reciprocal depression. Later when the S–T segment becomes normal the T waves invert. This pattern together with low voltage is also seen in constrictive pericarditis.

Pericarditis

In contrast to cardiac infarction, the current of injury of pericarditis usually involves the whole of the epicardium, so that S–T elevation is found in all leads without the reciprocal depression which is characteristic of the former. The T waves are initially low but upright and do not invert until the S–T segment has returned to the isoelectric level (Fig. 6.19b).

Ventricular aneurysms

The appearances resemble those of acute epicardial ischaemia but persist indefinitely.

Acute endocardial ischaemia

This produces horizontal or downward sloping depression of the S–T segment and may occur during an anginal attack, whether spontaneous or produced by an effort test. In the latter it is always best seen in leads V.4–6 (Fig. 6.20b).

Left ventricular hypertrophy

S–T depression occurs in the lead with the tallest R waves and in advanced cases is accompanied by T wave inversion.

Bundle branch block

S–T depression occurs in the leads with the tall slurred R waves together with inverted T waves.

Digitalis

This causes depression of the S–T segment beginning at its junction with the T waves and causing the segment to slope downwards. As the effect becomes more marked the T wave

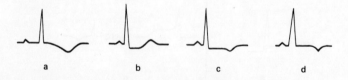

a   b   c   d

Fig. 6.20 S–T depression and T wave inversion. (a) Digitalis effect. The S–T segment slopes downward and the T wave becomes progressively smaller until it is invisible. (b) Acute sub-endocardial ischaemia. The S–T segment is depressed and horizontal or slopes downward. (c) Ventricular hypertrophy. In the early stages the pattern may resemble (b). Later there may also be T wave inversion (c) or T wave inversion may occur without S–T depression as in (d).

finally disappears. It is always best seen in the lead with the tallest R waves. The effect commonly persists for several days after Digitalis has been discontinued until the drug is completely eliminated (Fig. 6.20a).

Quinidine

This causes horizontal S–T depression leading to an upright wave, so-called 'roller-coaster' effect.

Abnormalities of the T waves

Abnormally tall T waves

These may occur in the first few hours of infarction and also when the intracellular potassium is abnormally high. They are

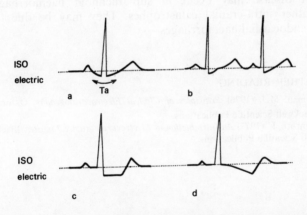

Fig. 6.21 Normal and abnormal cardiographic patterns after exercise. (a) and (b) show normal responses to exercise. In (A) the P–R segment is depressed due to the atrial T wave (TA) which continues into the S–T segment simulating S–T depression. In (b) there is depression beginning at the junction of the QRS with the S–T segment (the J Point). The S–T segment slopes upward and may merge imperceptibly into the T wave. In (c) and (d) the patterns are abnormal and indicate ischaemia. The segment is depressed and horizontal or slopes downward.

only indirectly related to the plasma potassium level.

Abnormally low or inverted T waves

These may be caused by ventricular hypertrophy, bundle branch block, myocardial ischaemia, and pericarditis. These have already been described under abnormalities of the S–T segment.

Low potassium

This lowers the terminal portion of the S–T segment, and the upstroke of the T wave which consequently develops a sinuous contour.

Intracranial lesions

Sharply pointed T waves resembling those of ischaemic heart disease may occur in sub-arachnoid haemorrhage or other intra-cranial catastrophes. They may be due to sub-endocardial haemorrhages.

FURTHER READING

Goldman, M.J. (1976) *Principles of Clinical Electrocardiography*. Oxford; Blackwell Scientific Publications.
Schamroth, L. (1977) *An Introduction to Electrocardiography*. Oxford: Blackwell Scientific Publications.

7. The Heart Rate and Rhythm and The Dysrhythmias

The average heart rate in healthy adults is about 72 per minute but ranges between 50 and 100 per minute. The average rate in women is about 10 beats per minute more and it is much faster in infants and young children. The lower ranges of normality are found in elderly subjects and in athletes, in whom the resting rate is commonly as low as 50 per minute. During sleep the average rate is commonly about 60 per minute. The heart slows physiologically in response to vagal stimulation; it may precede or accompany a vaso-vagal faint and occurs with raised intracranial pressure and sub-thyroidism. The heart is slowed by drugs producing beta-blockade, by Prenylamine and other drugs used in the treatment of hypertension. Acute pathological 'insults' to the heart such as cardiac infarction or cardiac catheterization may produce marked bradycardia or circulatory collapse due to cardiac standstill.

Tachycardia may occur physiologically due to increased sympathetic activity on emotion, when it commonly reaches 120 per minute, on maximum physical exercise or sexual intercourse when rates of 170 per minute may be reached. Tachycardia mediated by sympathetic activity is also a normal response to hyperthyroidism, pyrexia (an increase of 20 beats per minute per 1°C), oligaemia, 'shock', alcohol or heart failure. The tachycardia due to any of these causes persists for hours, days, or weeks, but only if it is due to emotion does the rate slow appreciably during sleep. In all of the instances mentioned the rhythm is perfectly regular and the jugular venous pressure, pulse and heart sounds are all normal. Carotid sinus pressure produces slight and gradual slowing but this is only temporary. Tachycardia also occurs in hypervolaemia whether due to pregnancy or chronic severe anaemia if the haemoglobin is below about 7 g per cent. In both these instances the venous pressure is commonly slightly raised and there is peripheral vaso-dilatation with a large pulse pressure.

When the heart rate exceeds about 110 per minute the cardiogram commonly shows junctional depression of the ST segment, sometimes as much as 2 or 3 mm below the iso-electric line. However, although the segment slopes upwards it is sometimes difficult to differentiate the appearance from that due to an ischaemic response to exercise (see Fig. 6.21, p. 97).

For the most part the heart rhythm is regular but in children, young adults and the elderly there is a phasic change with respiration called sinus arrhythmia—the heart accelerating during inspiration and slowing with expiration. This is usually abolished if the rate is increased by exercise or from other cause and this probably accounts for its rarity in the course of rheumatic fever. However, its presence does not exclude the possibility of rheumatic fever.

It has been thought that the heart rhythm remains regular apart from sinus arrhythmia and occasional ectopic beats throughout the 24 hours. However, it has now become possible to analyse continuous records over periods of 24 hours or more. It has been found that supraventricular tachycardia, junctional (nodal) rhythm and second degree heart block occur quite frequently in apparently normal subjects. Moreover, about 10 percent of such subjects showed dysrhythmias previously thought to have a serious significance. They included multifocal ventricular ectopic beats, sometimes occurring during the vulnerable repolarisation phase of the previous beat (R-on-T), short bouts of ventricular tachycardia and bigeminy. Further study of these occurrences and long-term follow up of the subjects showing them is clearly required to establish whether the subjects are truly normal and the dysrhythmias do not have the serious significance formerly attributed to them. Alternatively, a long-term follow up of a larger series may indicate that these dysrhythmias presage sudden death or indicate unsuspected heart disease.

Dysrhythmias (erroneously termed arrhythmias)

The term dysrhythmia is used to describe abnormalities of rate or rhythm due to the origin of impulses from an abnormal ectopic focus or to abnormal transmission of a normally arising impulse. The former include ectopic atrial or ventricular premature beats and tachycardias which may be paroxysmal or persistent. They may be supraventricular arising from the atrium or junctional (nodal) tissue or ventricular. More persistent tachycardias include atrial flutter and fibrillation. Abnormal conduction of a normally arising impulse produces the condition known as atrioventricular block which may be partial or complete.

Ectopic foci, re-entry and reciprocating rhythms

Consideration of these phenomena is fundamental to explanations of dysrhythmias. It has been shown that abnormal foci in the heart may produce isolated or rhythmic impulses disturbing the normal basic rhythm. They may occur apparently spontaneously or due to local anoxia. In any case depolarisation at the ectopic site is probably induced by a change in cell membrane permeability, allowing abnormal and unexpected depolarisation in the adjacent cells as described previously in the section on electrocardiography. The term re-entry is used to describe the return of an impulse to an area previously stimulated by the same impulse. The relative refractory period (p. 74) does not occur simultaneously throughout the heart muscle; some areas may be completely refractory while adjacent ones are not. An impulse will stimulate the latter and only activate the adjacent refractory zone after an interval, during which the originally stimulated zone may have recovered its excitability and respond a second time. (Fig. 7.1) Variations in the relative refractory period

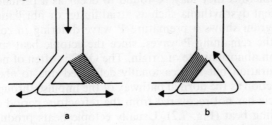

a   b

Fig. 7.1 Diagram of Re-entry. (a) The pathway of an impulse shown by the arrows avoids a refractory area (shaded). (b) After a brief interval the impulse can pass up the previously refractory area to stimulate the point of origin again and then retrace its original route. The process may be repeated indefinitely resulting in fibrillation.

from one area to another are particularly prone to occur with relative ischaemia or in patches of fibrosis. Return of the impulse to previously stimulated areas may be repeated endlessly so that unco-ordinated fibrillary contraction may occur at high speed. Re-entry in small areas of muscle (micro re-entry) leads in this way to fibrillation, and is much commoner in the atrium than in the ventricles. A long re-entrant pathway occurs if there is an accessory bundle of conducting tissue between the atrium and the ventricle as in the pre-excitation (Wolff-Parkinson-White) syndrome (p. 88). In the latter circumstance the impulse may pass to the ventricle by the normal route but then return retrogradely by the accessory pathway when its refractory period is over. The return of the impulse to the atrium produces a further atrial contraction and is followed by another descent via the normal AV route producing a so-called reciprocating paroxysmal tachycardia.

Atrial ectopic beats (atrial premature beats)

It should be noted that the commonly used expression extrasystole is inaccurate. The ectopic beat is premature but not supernumerary. It arises from the discharge of an ectopic focus anywhere in the right or left atrium often in healthy subjects for no apparent reason. Rarely they are provoked by irritation of the atrium by adjacent inflammatory conditions and occasionally by anoxia or electrolyte disturbance especially those associated with a low potassium. When they are numerous they may be found to occur as a prelude to a persistent dysrhythmia such as atrial flutter or fibrillation. A cardiogram shows a premature P wave differing in contour from the remaining P waves, since the ectopic beat spreads from an abnormal site of origin. The QRS is often of normal configuration but is occasionally deformed due to aberrant conduction as the normal pathway of the impulse through the ventricle has not recovered from the refractory period of the preceding beat (Fig. 7.2). Usually ectopic beats produce no symptoms but if they are frequent a sensation of fluttering may lead to anxiety. No treatment is required unless there is evident anoxia or electrolyte disturbance which should be corrected.

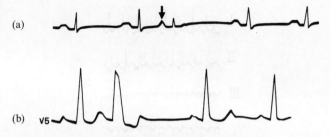

Fig. 7.2 (a) An atrial ectopic (premature) beat. The arrow indicates a premature abnormally shaped P wave indicating an origin in an ectopic focus. It is conducted to the ventricle producing a QRS of normal duration but its unusual shape indicates aberrant intraventricular conduction. The interval between the ectopic and the succeeding P wave is nearly normal so that three beats occupy nearly the normal time and the beat is not an 'extra-systole. (b) The second beat is premature. The QRS duration exceeds 0.12 sec and is not preceded by a P wave. It is a ventricular ectopic (premature) beat. As it shows a notched broad R wave in V5 it has arisen in the right ventricle.

Paroxysmal atrial tachycardia

Mechanism and cardiogram. In this condition impulses are produced from an ectopic focus in the atrium at rates ranging between 150 and 220 per minute. In some cases the mechanism may be a reciprocating tachycardia due to the presence of an accessory A–V pathway—the pre-excitation syndrome (p. 88). Since the impulse does not arise in the S–A node its spread across the atrium follows an abnormal pathway and the P waves are inverted or abnormal in contour. Sometimes they coincide with the ventricular complex and cannot be seen at all in conventional leads although they are always obvious in oesophageal or intra-atrial leads (Fig. 7.3). The QRS complexes are sometimes broadened due to functional bundle branch block brought about by the tachycardia and if at the same time the P waves cannot be discerned the appearance may be difficult to distinguish from ventricular tachycardia. However, such cases can usually be differentiated by the detection of P waves preceding each ventricular complex in the oesophageal or intra-atrial cardiogram (Fig. 7.4).

The dysrhythmia may complicate infections, surgical operations or heart disease of almost any kind, but it may occur in otherwise normal individuals in whom it may be provoked by violent exercise, strong tea or coffee, alcohol or even a sudden

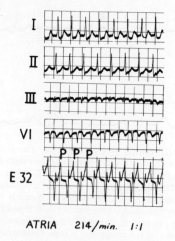

ATRIA 214/min. 1:1

Fig. 7.3 Paroxysmal tachycardia at a regular rate of 214 per min. The P waves can be seen only in the esophageal lead E32.

jolt. The onset is characteristically abrupt, the heart reaching a rate of 140 to 220 per minute within a few beats. It may persist at that speed for hours or days and is perfectly regular. The patient is often alarmed by this sensation of rapid fluttering in the chest, and may feel dizzy or unduly breathless on exertion. If the rate is very fast, there may be syncope or angina, especially if the attack is long-lasting or if there is associated heart disease. In such cases congestive failure or pulmonary oedema may result. In some cases frequency of micturition occurs, apparently through a reflex mechanism, depending on altered pressure-volume relationships in the atria, initiating a reflex arc through the autonomic nervous system. On examination rapid regular rhythm is often the only abnormal finding and the jugular pulse and heart sounds are normal. Carotid pressure either terminates the attack or is entirely without effect.

The attack can sometimes be terminated by physical manoeuvres such as placing the head between the knees, pressing on the carotid sinus or eyeballs, inducing retching or drinking iced water. Some patients discover bizarre methods of terminating the attack such as performing a handstand or by learning to perform the Valsalva manoeuvre in which they

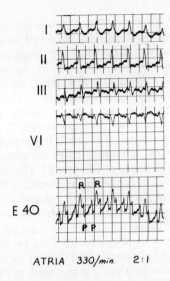

ATRIA 330/min.   2:1

Fig. 7.4 Supraventricular tachycardia with 2:1 A–V block and left bundle branch block. Two P waves for each R wave can be seen in the esophageal lead E40. 2:1 Atrial tachycardia is commonly due to digoxin intoxication.

forcibly attempt to expire against a closed glottis and with pinched nostrils. If these mechanical manoeuvres fail and the attack is incapacitating drugs may be needed. Sometimes simple sedation with diazepam (Valium) 5–10 mg may be all that is required. However, if there is serious intrinsic heart disease, or if the rate is very rapid and the attack long lasting so as to produce serious symptoms, it may be desirable to terminate the dysrhythmia without delay. A certain method of doing this is by applying DC shock (p. 117). This, of course, can only be done in hospital, and usually a light anaesthetic is required. If this presents difficulties or if the apparatus is not readily available digoxin is the treatment of choice for patients with heart disease. If possible it should not be given as a temporising measure with the intention of giving DC shock later because shock given after digoxin is liable to produce dangerous dysrhythmias or even ventricular fibrillation. The dose of digoxin for an average sized adult may be 0.5 mg 8–hourly by mouth or 0.75 to 1.0 mg well-diluted intravenously. A large number of drugs are now available in addition to digoxin and they are classified according to their main mode of action. Beta-blocking drugs are perhaps the most generally useful and practolol 10 mg intravenously is probably the most consistently effective. If the attack is known to be a reciprocating tachycardia due to the pre-excitation syndrome Verapamil is the drug of choice. For supraventricular tachycardias other drugs in groups 2, 3 and 4 in the classification and also disopyramide from group 1 are often successful. Doses of individual drugs are given in the alphabetical summary of drugs in Chapter 27. However, it must be remembered that each of the antidysrhythmic drugs depresses myocardial contractility to a varying degree. The consequent dangers of medication must therefore be weighed against that of the dysrhythmia which is a self-limiting condition and often remarkably well tolerated for long periods. The doses must therefore not be excessive and therapy should, if possible, be limited to not more than 2 drugs used in succession. The application of DC shock as a last resort after the use of several drugs in high doses is particularly dangerous.

Paroxysmal atrial tachycardia with 2:1 A–V block

The mechanism and cardiogram. This dysrhythmia is produced as in the one just described, by the regular discharge of impulses at a rate between 140 and 240 from an ectopic focus in one or other of the atria. The essential difference is the presence of A–V block which is usually 2:1. This may be difficult to discern in the cardiogram as alternate P waves may be buried in the QRS. The point exactly midway between two obvious P waves should be scrutinised for a deformity which may represent the hidden P wave. As usual, in supraventricular dysrhythmias, oesophageal or intracardiac leads usually reveal hidden P waves clearly (Fig. 7.4). The ventricular rate lies between 70 and 140 according to the atrial rate. The ventricular rate may change abruptly with carotid sinus pressure if it transiently increases the block.

Clinical features. The condition is most often due to digitalis intoxication the effects of which are often aggravated by low intracellular potassium which may not be reflected by the serum level. Heart disease is nearly always present and the dysrhythmia is rarely seen in otherwise healthy hearts. As the ventricular rate is only between 80 and 110 per minute, dizziness, breathlessness, angina and exacerbation of heart failure are not conspicuous. However digitalis intoxication makes the patient feel generally unwell, often with headache and anorexia, and the expected improvement in pre-existing heart failure does not occur. The persistence of a heart rate of about 100 to 120 per minute should lead to a careful search for hidden P waves in the cardiogram. Sometimes these are most easily demonstrated by taking a record during carotid sinus pressure, when a transient increase in block may reveal a hidden P wave.

Treatment. If digitalis has been given and is the probable cause, DC shock is absolutely contra-indicated. Potassium supplements should be given and the drugs of choice are intravenous practolol or propranolol by oral administration.

Junctional (nodal) ectopic beats

The term 'junctional' is preferable to 'nodal' as it is often impossible to be certain whether the focus is precisely within the A–V node, the margins of which are somewhat indefinite. The impulse produces a normal QRS complex and retrograde spread across the atrium results in an inverted P wave which may occur just before, within or after the QRS complex. If it is buried within it, it may be revealed by an oesophageal or an intracardiac electrocardiogram.

Junctional (nodal) rhythm

If the S–A node is depressed by vagal overactivity or drugs the A–V junctional tissue takes over the function of pacemaking. The heart rate is 40 to 60 per minute and the complexes are as described for junctional ectopic beats. A characteristic clinical sign is the occurrence of a regular bradycardia between 40 and 60 per minute with cannon waves in the jugular pulse accompanying every heart beat, because simultaneous contraction of atria and ventricles means that the A–V valves are closed when the atrium contracts. The condition is benign and usually self-limiting. No treatment is required.

Junctional (nodal) tachycardia

Mechanism and cardiogram. The dysrhythmia is produced by the regular discharge of impulses at 140 to 220 per minute from the junctional tissues. The complexes resemble those described in Junctional Rhythm above. The P waves are commonly invisible in conventional leads but are always detectable in oeseophageal or intracardiac leads.

Clinical features. The condition clinically resembles atrial tachycardia. Usually, though not invariably there is some associated disease. Regular cannon waves accompany each ventricular beat as in junctional rhythm but the rapid rate makes them less striking.

Treatment. Treatment is similar to that of atrial tachycardia.

Atrial flutter

Mechanism and cardiogram. The mechanism of this dysrhythmia remains controversial. It was originally thought to depend on a re-entry mechanism which produced a wave of excitation following a circular re-entry pathway around the orifices of the venae cavae and spreading from there to both atria, the frequency ranging from 200 to 400 per minute. Studies with high speed cinematography suggested that the dysrhythmia was due to discharge of a single ectopic focus at this rate. At the present time research is tending to support the original theory of re-entry. A cardiogram shows a characteristic distortion of the base line to produce a 'saw-tooth' pattern of precise symmetry (Fig. 7.5). The peaks commonly occur at a rate of 300 per minute. The continuous oscillation of the base line was held to support the 'circus' movement theory because it suggested that a portion of the atria was being activated at every instant; however, it can equally be argued that the continuous oscillation is due to the atrial T waves filling the intervals between the peaks. The cardiographic distinction of flutter from paroxysmal atrial tachycardia, which is thought to be due to a single ectopic focus, is not sharp. In both conditions a continuous oscillation of the baseline can usually be found in at least one lead though that lead may be intra-atrial or oeseophageal. However, it remains true that an obvious 'saw-tooth' appearance in leads 2 and 3 with peaks called 'f' (for flutter) waves occurring between 200 or 400 per minute is associated with fairly constant clinical features described below and justifies the distinction of this dysrhythmia from atrial tachycardia. The ventricles usually respond to every third f wave but sometimes to every second

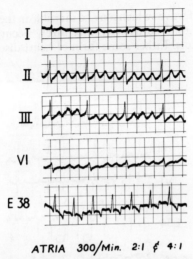

ATRIA 300/Min. 2:1 & 4:1

Fig. 7.5 Atrial Flutter. The symmetrical saw-tooth appearance in leads 2 and 3 is characteristic. The ventricular rate is regular at 75/min in the limb leads and 150/min in the esophageal lead E38 due to a change from 4:1 to 2:1 block.

or rarely to every fourth f wave. Such 3:1 or 4:1 response is rare in the group customarily termed paroxysmal atrial tachycardia. A further distinguishing feature is the slight variation in the interval between the peak of the f wave and the QRS complex. The ventricular rate is regular for considerable periods. It may abruptly change by simple multiples, as for example from 100 per minute to 150 per minute or 75 per minute as the A–V block changes from the common 3:1 to 2:1 or 4:1 (Fig. 7.5). A persistent unexplained regular tachycardia of 100 or 150 per minute should arouse suspicion of atrial flutter and this can commonly be diagnosed with confidence at the bedside by observing the response to carotid pressure. This may produce temporary ventricular standstill or increase the A–V block from the common 2:1 to 3:1 or even 4:1, causing an abrupt change in ventricular rate from 150 to 100 or 75 per minute. The original rate is abruptly resumed on release of carotid pressure and this is rare in any other dysrhythmia. It is advantageous to perform the manoeuvre while recording lead 2 so as to obtain a permanent record of the f waves which may be invisible in the conventional leads (Fig. 7.6). The dysrhythmia rarely occurs in perfectly healthy subjects. Either some form of heart disease is present

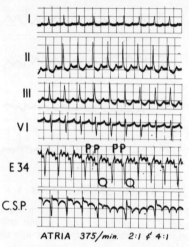

ATRIA 375/min. 2:1 & 4:1

Fig. 7.6 The conventional leads show a regular supraventricular tachycardia of 150/min without visible P or f waves. However these are visible in the esophageal lead E34 with a 2:1 block and carotid sinus pressure (CSP) produces the appearance of flutter with 2:1 and 4:1 block.

or there may be disease in any system of the body. In the latter case the underlying cause may be quite obscure and may finally prove to be a hidden neoplasm, a low grade infection, anaemia, thyrotoxicosis, or a painless episode of cardiac ischaemia. The condition is also common after any form of surgery and may be an annoying sequel to an otherwise successful closure of an atrial septal defect. The patient may complain of palpitations, effort dyspnoea due to a change of the A–V block on exercise to produce a ventricular rate of 150. If the dysrthythmia persists failure may occur in the presence ot serious underlying heart disease. Treatment with DC shock is almost invariably effective and only a very low energy of 50 W/sec is required. At this low level a general anaesthetic is not needed and the procedure can be performed with 10 mg of intravenous diazepam. Among the anti-dysrhythmic drugs digoxin, practolol, propranolol and disopyramide will sometimes restore sinus rhythm but DC shock is so much more dependable that it should be the first choice. Atrial flutter is an exasperating dysrhythmia for, although it is easy to convert to sinus rhythm, it has a strong tendency to recur if the underlying cause is not removed. This may be a more or less irremediable form of heart disease but it may also recur repeatedly following a completely successful closure of an atrial septal defect. In such cases, long-term administration of disopyramide, quinidine, in the form of kinidin durules, or digoxin may prevent recurrences.

Atrial fibrillation

Mechanism and cardiogram. It is now thought that this dysrhythmia may be initiated by the discharge of a single ectopic focus but that it is perpetuated by a micro re-entry mechanism. This produces waves of excitation circulating irregularly around the orifices of the venae cavae, and spreading in disorderly fashion across the atria to produce ineffectual fibrillary contractions. The cardiogram shows (f) waves at a rate between 300 and 500 per minute, (commonly 350/min) with an irregular ventricular response of 100-200/min. Characteristically, the f waves vary continuously in amplitude and frequency so that some resemble the saw-tooth appearance of atrial flutter while others are almost invisible (Fig. 7.7).

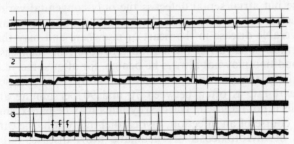

Fig. 7.7 Atrial Fibrillation. The f waves are variable in amplitude and frequency sometimes disappearing altogether. The ventricular response is irregular and slow due to digoxin.

In cases in which there is little variation in the f waves and the ventricular response is nearly regular between 100 and 180/

min the appearances closely resemble those of atrial flutter. Indeed, there is no sharp dividing line between the two conditions. Cases in which the f waves are predominantly tall and broad (coarse fibrillation) are often of recent onset and may be easily converted with DC shock to sinus rhythm. By contrast cases in which the f waves are small, irregular and at times invisible, often have long-standing fibrillation, with gross atrial enlargement and are frequently resistant to conversion. The pathology of the S–A node in atrial fibrillation is variable and only about half the cases show damage to the central specialized automatic cells and to the neuroganglia. Sometimes there is evidence of old pericarditis in the vicinity of the node. It should be noted that a patchy fibrosis of the atrium sometimes is found in chronic rheumatic heart disease and is the ideal basis for re-entry as the fibrotic areas delay and divert the passage of the impulse allowing adjacent areas to recover from their refractory period, and become responsive to a returning stimulus.

Clinical features. The commonest associations of the dysrhythmia are mitral valve disease and hyperthyroidism. It occurs in about 5–10 per cent of cases of ischaemic heart disease and a similar proportion of cases of hypertensive heart disease in whom it does not necessarily indicate associated coronary disease. It may complicate almost any form of heart disease but atrial septal defect is the only congenital variety in which it occurs. It may also be found in the absence of any discoverable disease in the heart or elsewhere and may then be termed 'lone' atrial fibrillation. However, in such cases the condition may not always be benign, for after some years heart failure may occur quite unaccountably. In this variety the heart rate is often between 70 and 90 per minute and digitalis is not required. The dysrhythmia may be paroxysmal in the course of an infection, myocardial infarction, the early stages of thyrotoxicosis or rheumatic heart disease, but it is more often permanent. The patient does not always notice palpitations at the onset but some degree of dyspnoea is usual. The deleterious effect on the circulation depends partly on the loss of atrial transport which may reduce the cardiac output by as much as 25 per cent and partly to the shortening of diastole due to the tachycardia which further reduces ventricular filling. In mitral stenosis there is already a mechanical obstruction to filling, and the summation of these factors produces a drastic fall in cardiac output and rise in left atrial and pulmonary venous pressure. This causes turgidity of the lungs with consequent dyspnoea and finally pulmonary oedema. Additional serious consequences of the low output in mitral stenosis are a tendency to venous thrombosis leading to pulmonary emboli, and left atrial thrombosis causing systemic emboli with perhaps a disastrous hemiplegia. In other forms of heart disease the effects of atrial fibrillation are not quite as serious and their severity depends to a considerable extent on the ventricular rate, which is always a major determinant of cardiac output.

Treatment. Since atrial fibrillation must usually be regarded as a permanent dysrhythmia the prime objects of treatment are control of the ventricular rate and prevention of emboli. The former is achieved by prompt digitalization (p. 295) and the latter by equally prompt introduction of permanent anti-coagulant therapy with heparin and warfarin (p. 298 and 306).

In cases in which the cause of atrial fibrillation has been removed or ameliorated, conversion to sinus rhythm can be attempted with DC shock. Thus it is reasonable to try it following a satisfactory mitral valvotomy or cure of hyperthyroidism, and it can also be considered if it is felt that the dysrhythmia is premature in an individual case of mitral disease, perhaps owing to an intercurrent infection, pregnancy or a surgical operation.

Conversion to sinus rhythm is not very often achieved in cases of 'lone' atrial fibrillation and when it is achieved it is often short-lived, perhaps because the dysrhythmia is due to an intrinsic disorder of the S–A node. For this reason conversion is only recommended in 'lone' atrial fibrillation if the patient has been informed of these possibilities but feels that possible relief of slight effort dyspnoea and return to normality outweighs them.

Finally it is emphasised that DC shock is more likely to be permanently successful if the dysrhythmia is of recent onset, the patient is relatively young, the 'f' waves in the cardiogram are coarse, and causative factors have been ameliorated or removed.

Ventricular ectopic (premature) beats

Mechanism and cardiogram. A ventricular ectopic or premature beat is produced by spontaneous depolarisation of a focus in either ventricle. A wave of depolarisation spreads from the focus through the ventricular muscle without passing down the bundle branches or through the Purkinje network. The impulse therefore produces a cardiographic pattern resembling that of bundle branch block (Fig. 7.2). An ectopic beat arising in the right ventricle produces an appearance resembling left bundle branch block; a left ventricular ectopic produces an appearance of a right bundle branch block but neither are preceded by P waves. The precise configuration of the QRS complex depends on the position in the ventricle of the ectopic focus, so that the cardiogram shows whether ectopics arise in the right or left ventricle and are derived from single or multiple foci. This is of some importance because left ventricular multifocal ectopics are more likely to lead to ventricular tachycardia or fibrillation.

If a sinus beat is regularly followed by a ventricular ectopic

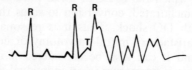

Fig. 7.8 An R–on–T Premature beat and Ventricular Fibrillation. A premature beat occurring during the T wave of the preceding beat (R–on–T) finds the muscle in various stages of refractoriness (the Relative Refractory Period). This is the essential pre-requisite for re-entry and ventricular fibrillation results, indicated by continuous large amplitude oscillations of the base-line irregular in amplitude and frequency.

beat the condition is known as 'coupling' and is common in digitalis intoxication though it may occur in health. If an ectopic beat occurs during the T wave of the previous sinus beat (the R-on-T phenomenon) ventricular fibrillation may occur through re-entry (Fig. 7.1 and 7.8). Ventricular fibrillation produces no effective contraction and the cardiac output falls to zero with potentially fatal results.

Ventricular ectopic beats may occur in normal individuals or in any form of heart disease. They may be provoked by digitalis and if coupling is present it should arouse suspicion of overdosage. Occurring during or after cardiac infarction, they may presage ventricular tachycardia or fibrillation and if they are frequent or multifocal they should be suppressed with Lignocaine (p. 299).

Ventricular tachycardia

Mechanism and cardiogram. There is a rapid discharge of impulses at 140–220 per minute from a single ectopic focus in one or other ventricle. The QRS complex is broad exceeding 0.12 seconds in duration and resembles that of bundle branch block as explained for unifocal ectopic beats. The T waves are opposite in direction to the R waves. The rhythm is almost regular and the R–R intervals vary by only 0.03 sec (Fig. 7.9). P waves occur independently at a slower rate, usually about 80 to 100 per minute and are best seen in intra-atrial or oesophageal records.

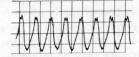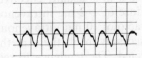

Fig. 7.9 Ventricular Tachycardia. The QRS complexes are widened beyond 0.12 sec. There is a regular tachycardia of 210/min and P waves cannot be seen so that the diagnosis of ventricular tachycardia is presumptive. A supraventricular tachycardia with hidden P waves and bundle branch block is a possibility.

Clinical features. The dysrhythmia very rarely occurs in healthy hearts but is common in cardiac infarction and it also occurs as a result of digitalis overdosage. Acidosis is an important contributory factor. The onset is abrupt and the ventricular rate is usually between 140 and 220 per minute. The attack may last for minutes, hours or even days. If the dysrhythmia occurs in seriously diseased hearts, symptoms of breathlessness, angina, faintness and hypotension commonly result. Since the atria and ventricles are contracting independently occasional atrial contractions occur against a closed A–V valve to produce a cannon' wave in the neck. The combination of slow, irregular 'cannon' waves with rapid regular ventricular action suggests the correct diagnosis. The perpetual variation of the P–R interval may cause a variation of intensity of the first heart sound, and in the presence of a regular tachycardia points to the diagnosis. Carotid pressure does not influence the tachycardia.

Differentiation from supraventricular tachycardia with bundle branch block depends upon the demonstration of independent P waves occurring at a slower rate than the QRS complex. Intra-atrial or oesophageal electrocardiograms are usually needed to demonstrate them.

Treatment. The dysrhythmia is a dangerous one, usually occurring in seriously ill patients and it must be promptly treated. Provided there is no suspicion of digitalis intoxication and facilities are readily to hand, DC shock is the method of choice (p. 117). Alternatively, Lignocaine 1 mg/kg in saline intravenously as a bolus followed by 1–2 mg/min in a 5 per cent glucose drip is usually effective. Alternatives are propranolol in a dose of 1–2 mg intravenously (occasionally up to 5 mg) or practolol 10 mg intravenously may be used. The prospect of success with all these methods is increased if acidosis is corrected. The tendency to recurrence may be minimised by continuing the Lignocaine infusion for 24 or 48 hours and then substituting propranolol 40 to 80 mg 8–hourly by mouth. If the dysrhythmia was caused by cardiac infarction this prophylaxis should be continued for a year.

Ventricular fibrillation

Mechanism and cardiogram. This potentially lethal dysrhythmia is caused by a re-entry mechanism (Fig. 7.8). Irregular disorderly repetitive activation throughout the muscle produces fibrillary twitching without effective contraction. As a result the cardiac output falls to zero, consciousness is lost and death follows quickly if resuscitation is not effective, or effective ventricular contraction does not return spontaneously as in complete A–V block.

Clinical features. Ventricular fibrillation commonly occurs as a result of coronary thrombosis or cardiac infarction and may be the terminal event in many forms of heart disease. It may be caused by drugs and electrolyte disturbances, and the combination of potassium depletion and digoxin over-dosage is particularly dangerous. It may be the cause of death in electrocution and drowning and the cause of some of the syncopal attacks in complete A–V block. The latter is probably one of the few conditions in which ventricular fibrillation may be transient.

Treatment. The dysrhythmia causes complete cessation of the circulation and death occurs unless effective resuscitation is applied within three minutes (p. 285). The crucial procedure is defibrillation by DC shock described below. This should be effected with the least possible delay and external cardiac massage and mouth to mouth respiration should be instantly applied, and continued until a DC shock can be given. The correction of acidosis and the other measures described in Chapter 25 are vital.

Direct current (DC) shock

Theory

The application of an electrical shock of suitable energy to the chest results in depolarisation of all the cardiac muscle cells. The energy level must be sufficient to do this but not enough to damage the skin or body as a whole. The most effective method is the use of high energy for an extremely brief time—far shorter than a 60 Hz alternating current would allow. The usual levels required range from 50 W/sec to 400 W/sec.

Technique. Flutter rarely requires an energy level exceeding 50 W/sec and this can be given under the light sedation produced by 5–10 mg of intravenous diazepam (Valium). High energy levels necessitate a brief anaesthetic unless the patient is unconscious from ventricular fibrillation. Elective dc shock treatment is therefore performed on a fasting patient appropriately sedated or anaesthetised. The patient is placed on his side with the left shoulder uppermost and electrode jelly is vigorously rubbed into the skin of the second right intercostal space and over the angle of the left scapula. Most instruments are capable of recording the cardiogram through the electrodes used for applying the shock and the rhythm should be monitored and recorded before and after each shock. The instrument is charged to the desired energy setting and synchronised to discharge just after the R wave of the cardiogram so as to avoid the vulnerable relative refractory period. After a test discharge, the operator, wearing rubber gloves, holds the electrodes firmly in the positions mentioned. The energy level selected depends on the dysrhythmia and the clinical circumstances. Atrial flutter almost always responds to 50 W/sec while the desperate emergency of ventricular fibrillation should be treated immediately with 350 W/sec to avoid the delay of repeated unsuccessful attempts. The frequency of complications increases considerably above levels of 250 W/sec and this should therefore be the starting level for all other conditions. The maximum energy applied should not exceed 400 W/sec and three or four attempts can be made if immediate success is not achieved. The blood pressure and cardiogram should be monitored continuously for the first 15 minutes and then at intervals for two hours. If the procedure was an elective one, the patient can then usually be allowed to go home.

Failure and complications. In a proportion of cases the attempt at conversion is unsuccessful. This is common in patients with advanced heart disease, 'lone' atrial fibrillation or serious mitral disease. Both the incidence of atrial fibrillation and its resistance to conversion increase with the age of the patient. Complications are commonest if shocks exceeding 250 W/sec are used and include elevation of cardiac enzymes, pulmonary oedema, hypotension, T wave abnormalities in the cardiogram, systemic embolism and an audible third heart sound. A rise in the serum enzymes seems to have little clinical significance but pulmonary oedema may be serious. This may be caused by the resumption of normal activity of the right atrium with failure of the left to contract satisfactorily despite the presence of P waves. Treatment with intermittent venous occlusion and intravenous diuretics (p. 11) is usually successful. Hypotension usually recovers spontaneously. Embolism is rare but 10 days preliminary anticoagulation is advisable in subjects with mitral valve disease, and in others who have a history of days or weeks of uncontrolled tachycardia which may have led to a low cardiac output and fresh venous thrombosis. DC shock is often followed by transient but relatively benign dysrhythmias such as bradycardia with nodal or ventricular escape or multiple premature beats which rarely give rise to anxiety. Serious dysrhythmias including ventricular tachycardia or ventricular fibrillation may occur if digoxin has not been stopped for 24 or 48 hours before the procedure. If they do occur they can sometimes be converted by a further shock or treatment with Lignocaine, propranolol, or disopyramide.

Nomenclature. Various bizarre, inappropriate, ugly or inaccurate terms have been used to describe this method of treatment, including cardioversion, electroversion, countershock, and defibrillation (mercifully not deflutter); it is apparent that none of them is either necessary or appropriate.

FURTHER READING

Clarke, Joan, M., Hamer, J., Shelton, J.R., Taylor, Sue, Venning, G.R. (1976) The rhythm of the normal human heart, *Lancet*, **2**, 508.

Stock, J.P.P. & Williams, D.O. (1974) *Diagnosis and Treatment of Cardiac Arrhythmias* London: Butterworths.

8. Disorders of Conduction

Sinus standstill, sino-atrial block and the 'Sick Sinus Syndrome'
Mechanism and cardiogram. In sino-atrial standstill the sino-atrial node capriciously fails to produce an impulse, causing periods of complete standstill of variable length. In sino-atrial block it seems that an impulse must be generated in the sino-atrial node that is not transmitted to the atrium, for the period of standstill in the cardiogram equals 2 P–P intervals (Fig. 8.1).

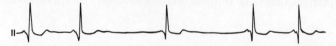

Fig. 8.1 Sino-Atrial Block. A P wave is missing between the 2nd and 3rd and 3rd and 4th beats. The prolonged P–P intervals are exactly twice the length of the other P–P intervals. This suggests that an impulse was produced in the S–A node at the expected time but block prevented it from emerging to the atrial muscle to produce a P wave (The potentials within the S–A node are always too small to appear in conventional leads). The next impulse occurs after the expected interval and passes into the atrial muscle to produce a P wave in normal fashion.

Both of these phenomena may be produced by digoxin or the anti-dysrhythmic drugs. They may, however, be due to the disease of the S–A node as part of the 'sick sinus syndrome', which seems to be due to a primary fibrosis of the S–A node. There is usually persistent bradycardia in addition to the sino-atrial block and episodes of sinus arrest. The P–P intervals may be long enough to give a rate of about 40 per minute and thus allow the A–V node to 'escape' producing QRS complexes of normal duration without a preceding P wave. The predominant bradycardia may be interrupted by paroxysms of supraventricular tachycardia of varying duration. The condition appears to be due to an intrinsic disease of the S–A node which may be fibrotic.

Clinical features. The condition occurs chiefly in elderly subjects in whom the bradycardia may cause dizziness, syncope, weakness, lack of energy and effort dyspnoea because the heart cannot adequately increase its cardiac output by increase of stroke volume. The episodes of tachycardia may result in palpitations, dizziness and effort dyspnoea because shortened diastole reduces filling and output.

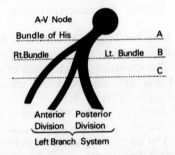

Fig. 8.2 The A–V node, Bundle of His and Bundle Branches and the effect of interruption of conduction at various levels. Interruption of the anterior division of the left bundle produces left anterior hemiblock (Fig. 8.3). Interruption of the posterior division of the left bundle is rare. Interruption of the right bundle produces right bundle branch block (p. 93). Interruption of the right bundle and left anterior division produces right bundle branch block with left anterior hemiblock (Fig. 8.3). Interruption of the left bundle produces left bundle branch block (p. 93). Interruption of the Bundle of His (above level A) produces complete A–V block with narrow QRS<0.12 sec because an idioventricular impulse can pass normally down the bundle branches. Interruption of the Bundle of His between A and B blocks left and right bundle branches (bi-fascicular block) causing complete A–V block with wide QRS>0.12 sec. Interruption below level of (C) produces trifascicular complete A–V block with wide QRS>0.12 sec. This is the commonest type of permanent complete A–V block.

Treatment. The alternation of tachycardia and bradycardia demands treatment with a pacemaker (p.127) to maintain a rate of 70/min together with an anti-dysrhythmic drug such as propranolol or disopyramide to prevent paroxysms of tachycardia. Treated in this way the condition seems relatively benign though a few patients develop complete A–V block. The majority, who are elderly at onset, live for more than five years. However, the condition is but newly described and prognosis is not yet thoroughly known.

Intraventricular block

The reader is advised to study Figure. 8.2 before reading this section.

Bundle branch block (p. 93 for cardiographic features), may be functional or organic due to ischaemic or idiopathic fibrosis or calcification or associated with dilatation and hypertrophy.

Left anterior hemi-block. This condition is due to interruption or failure of function of the anterior fascicle of the left bundle branch. The sequence of activation of the ventricle is consequently altered and this produces abnormal left axis deviation exceeding $-30°$ (Fig. 8.3).

Left posterior hemi-block. This rare variety is due to interruption or malfunction of the multiple posterior fascicles of the left bundle. The altered sequence of activation results in abnormal right axis deviation.

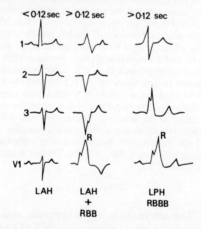

Fig. 8.3 Left anterior hemiblock (LAH) is shown by the dominant S in lead 2 indicating left axis exceeding minus 30°. Left anterior hemiblock with Right bundle branch block (LAH + RBB) is indicated by RSR' exceeding 0.12 sec in V.1. with dominant S in lead 2. Left posterior hemiblock with Right bundle branch block (LPH + RBBB) is indicated by RSR' > 0.12 second and marked right axis deviation.

Right bundle branch block with left anterior hemi-block. This is indicated by the combination of the right branch block pattern in V1 together with left axis deviation exceeding −30°C (Fig. 8.3). Complete A–V block inevitably follows if the left posterior fascicles become involved.

Right bundle branch block with left posterior hemi-block. This is a very unusual combination of the right branch block appearance in V1 with abnormal right axis in the limb leads. Complete A–V block follows if the anterior division of the left branch becomes diseased as well.

Atrio-ventricular block

Definition. Atrio-ventricular (A–V) block means partial or complete failure of transmission of the impulse from the atrium to the ventricle.

Types. These are often spoken of as first degree, second degree and third degree or complete block, although the condition infrequently passes from one degree to another. In partial block (1st degree) there is simply delay in transmission through the A–V junctional tissues resulting in prolongation of the P–R interval beyond the normal upper limit of 0.21 secs in adults. In so-called second degree heart block, occasional atrial beats are not transmitted. Sometimes there is progressive prolongation of the P–R interval until a beat is dropped, following which the sequence begins again with the shortest P–R interval of the series (Fig. 8.5). This is the Wenckebach phenomenon or Mobitz type 1 block. In other cases there are simply capricious failures of transmission of the atrial beat without preceding sequential prolongation of the P–R interval. This is sometimes known as Mobitz—type II. Any of these varieties occasionally occur in normal individuals or they may be due to drugs, such as digoxin, or beta-blockers, rheumatic fever and ischaemic heart disease.

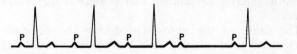

Fig. 8.4 The Wenckebach phenomenon. There is a progressive lengthening of the P–R interval until a P wave fails to produce a ventricular response. The next P wave produces a ventricular response with a normal P–R interval.

The varieties with dropped beats occasionally progress to complete A–V block, indicating an organic cause. In complete A–V block none of the atrial impulses is conducted to the ventricle, so that the atria may be activated normally by P waves at a rate between 70 and 100 per minute while the ventricles are activated by a pacemaker in the His-Purkinje system at a rate between 40 and 60 per minute. Sometimes in complete A–V block the atria fibrillate or flutter and the ventricles are activated at an idioventricular rhythm from a pacemaker in the His-Purkinje system as described. This variety can be caused by digitalis but more often the pathology is as described below.

Pathology. The possible sites of lesions causing complete heart block are shown in Figure 8.2. Permanent complete A–V block is rarely due to ischaemic heart disease. The commonest cause is an idiopathic fibrosis affecting the right bundle and both the anterior and posterior divisions of the left bundle—a tri-fascicular block. This is occasionally preceded by right bundle block and left anterior hemi-block with A–V conduction depending on the posterior fascicles of left division. The first part of the bundle of His passes through the fibrous part of the interventricular septum and is in close relationship to the aortic valve. Calcification may spread from the valve to the bundle resulting in a mono-fascicular block. Cardiac infarction does not usually result in permanent complete A–V block; the A–V node and the bundle of His are supplied by a branch of the right coronary artery so that a posterior infarction can be accompanied by a temporary complete A–V block. But infarction of the atrium does not occur and the block due to transient ischaemia usually recovers in a few days. However, if the right branch and both fascicles of the left are involved in an extensive septal infarct, complete heart block occurs and is usually fatal, as there is usually occlusion of both anterior descending and posterior interventricular arteries.

The cause of the fibrosis producing the common tri-fascicular type of complete A–V block is unknown. Long ago the author suggested that it might be due to auto-immune disease and this possibility is still under investigation. Rarely complete A–V block occurs as a congenital anomaly, either alone or associated with a ventricular septal defect. It may follow surgical closure of any of the varieties of ventricular septal defect, and sometimes occurs in cardiomyopathies and reticulosis involving the heart.

Clinical features. In the common idiopathic variety the patients are usually between 70 and 90 years of age and give no history suggestive of ischaemic heart disease. They are often lethargic, weak and breathless, but attribute this to old age. A dramatic syncopal attack may be the first symptom and may be due to temporary failure of the idioventricular pacemaker causing standstill or to a brief episode of ventricular fibrillation. A short attack causes only momentary dizziness, but if ventricular fibrillation or standstill lasts more than 5–10 seconds the patient falls to the ground sometimes with convulsions, incontinence or injury. There is deathly pallor and no palpable pulse until a bright flush indicates resumption of cardiac output and flooding of the dilated skin vessels. Unconsciousness rarely lasts more than about 30 seconds and recovery may be accelerated by deliberate thumps over the heart. The patient may have noticed oedema due to congestive failure and occasionally there are attacks of ischaemic cardiac pain at rest, lasting for 15–45 minutes. The explanation of these is uncertain for although they may be accompanied by bizarre deeply inverted T waves, the serum enzymes do not rise, and the clinical condition does not deteriorate. They may be associated with phases of excessive bradycardia. The clinical signs in complete heart block are striking. The patient is often sluggish, apathetic, and sometimes a little confused. The heart rate is regular, between 40 and 60 per minute, and there are irregular cannon waves in the jugular pulse (Fig. 2.6). The arterial pulse has a 'water-hammer' quality due to the large stroke volume and there may be capillary pulsation. The blood pressure is often of the order of 230/70 mmHg. The dissociation of atrial from ventricular activity causes perpetual variation of the P–R interval, with consequent variation of the intensity of the first heart sound which occasionally has a booming quality—'cannon sound' (p. 32). Varied intensity of the first sound with regular rhythm is diagnostic of heart block. The first sounds are quiet when the P–R interval is either too short to open the A–V valve fully or so long that the A–V valve has almost closed on the rising tide of blood in the ventricle (see Fig. 2.9). There is often a loud mid-systolic murmur at the base of the heart due to the large stroke volume but in some cases it is due to calcific aortic stenosis—the causative lesion of the block.

Radiology. There is often considerable cardiac enlargement due to the large stroke volume. However, this is not the sole explanation as some enlargement often persists following satisfactory pacing. Sometimes there are signs of heart failure with hilar congestion and pleural effusions.

The cardiogram. There are regular P waves between 70 and 100 per minute with independent ventricular complexes at a rate between 40 and 60/min. The duration of the QRS complexes depends on the site of the block and the position of the ventricular pacemaker. If the block is high the impulse may arise above the bifurcation of the bundle of His so that intraventricular conduction follows a normal pathway, the QRS duration is less than 0.12 sec, and has a normal configuration (Fig. 8.5a). If the block is below the bifurcation, the idioventricular impulse cannot follow normal pathways and the QRS duration exceeds 0.12 sec (Fig. 8.5b). This is the usual finding in the common idiopathic variety of permanent complete A–V block.

Prognosis. 'First degree heart block' is usually transient and when it persists seems to have no serious significance. The Mobitz Type I variety of partial heart block is also benign

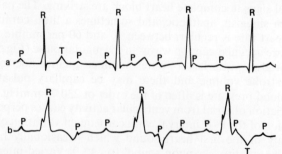

Fig. 8.5 Complete A–V Block. (a) With normal QRS complexes < 0.12 sec and therefore due to monofascicular block. (b) With widened QRS complexes > 0.12 sec and therefore due to bifascicular or trifascicular block.

and may even occur rarely in normal subjects. The Mobitz Type II block sometimes progresses to 2:1, 3:1 or complete heart block due to fibrosis of both bundle branches. In such cases there is considerable risk of sudden death in the days or weeks following the first Stokes-Adams attack. However, if these are survived syncopal attacks usually diminish in frequency and the patient may live for many years. However, death eventually ensues either from a fatal Stokes-Adams attack or from congestive failure. The prognosis has been greatly improved by the use of pacemakers which enable the patient to live for many years.

A–V block occurring during the course of inferior cardiac infarction raises the mortality to about 50 per cent, but this has been somewhat reduced by prompt treatment with pacemakers. If the first few days are survived the heart block usually disappears and the prognosis follows the ordinary pattern for cardiac infarction (p. 169). Complete block complicating anteroseptal infarction is a disastrous event. The block usually implies occlusion of both anterior and posterior arteries of the septum and the infarct is very extensive. The patient usually dies in spite of pacing.

Treatment. First degree heart block requires no treatment. In second degree heart block a pacemaker is indicated if the condition is unstable and syncopal attacks indicate episodes of complete block. Long-acting oral isoprenaline is insufficiently dependable for prolonged treatment and since the first Stoke-Adams attack could prove fatal it is wise to forestall it by the introduction of a pacemaker. With careful supervision these are now thoroughly dependable and can be implanted for permanent complete block with the confident expectation that they will transform the patients' life. He may be changed from a housebound, sluggish, partially confused individual, threatened with dangerous syncopal attacks, to an alert, relatively vigorous self-sufficient person.

A temporary pacemaker as a rule should be inserted immediately on diagnosis of persistent complete block. The usual procedure is to pass an electrode through an antecubital vein to the apex of the right ventricle where it is wedged. The proximal end is connected to a pacemaker at the patient's bedside. A 'demand' pacemaker is used which provides an impulse whenever their heart rate drops below a predetermined rate of about 70 per min. This usually produces prompt improvement in the patient's condition and after 5 or 7 days a permanent system can be introduced. The electrode is passed from a jugular vein to the right ventricle, and under a general anaesthetic, its proximal end is passed through a subcutaneous tunnel to the axilla or upper abdominal wall where the permanent pacemaker battery is implanted. The temporary system is then removed. It is not uncommon for the endocardial electrode to become dislodged once or twice during the first seven days during which close observation is essential. If, despite repeated attempts a stable position is not found an electrode is sutured to the epicardium through a small thoracotomy. By either method, pacing is then usually trouble free for two or three years until renewal of the battery is required. Frequently no adjuvant medication is needed but occasionally failure persists despite satisfactory pacing and requires digoxin and diuretics. In some subjects pacing is followed by the return of sinus rhythm and to avoid 'competition' between the artificial and physiological pacemakers for control of the ventricle, a 'demand' pacemaker is used which supplies an impulse only if the R–R interval falls below a value giving a heart rate of 70 per minute. Careful follow up of patients with pacemakers is essential and they should attend a special clinic organised for electronic testing as well as medical supervision at three-monthly intervals. The patient is seen monthly by his practitioner and told to report sooner if there is any change in heart rate. If these precautions are meticulously observed pacing is a thoroughly satisfactory method of treatment which prolongs the patient's life and vastly improves its quality.

FURTHER READING

Pacemakers (1972) Symposium including pacing for Chronic Rhythm Disorders and in cardiac infarction; complications and follow-up. *Progress in Cardiovascular Disease*, **14**(5).

9. High Blood Pressure

Definition

Ideally an abnormal blood pressure should be defined in terms of peripheral vascular resistance and a value exceeding 25 units (p. 47) due to arteriolar narrowing is abnormal. However, this is inconvenient clinically as the cardiac output can rarely be measured at the same time as the blood pressure and the latter alone must therefore be used. A value of 140/90 mmHg is usually considered to be the upper limit of normal. For although it is recognised that the average blood pressure tends to rise smoothly and steadily with age and there is no sharp level at which an abnormal mechanism can always be found, a pressure of 140/90 mmHg marks an upper limit above which the risk of serious complications caused by a raised pressure sharply increases. It is therefore clinically expedient both from the point of view of prognosis and treatment to accept this as the upper limit of normality.

Causes and types

In the majority of cases no single cause is found for an abnormally high blood pressure and the condition has been called benign essential hypertension on the assumption that the high blood pressure is an essential component of the biological constitution of the patient. It has been pointed out however that the condition is neither benign nor essential and that this is a serious misnomer. It is simply called high blood pressure of unknown cause, in this classification:

1. High blood pressure of unknown cause
2. High blood pressure secondary to:
   i. renal disease: (a) glomerulo-nephritis (b) hydro-nephrosis (c) polycystic disease (d) renal artery stenosis (e) pyelonephritis

ii. Endocrine disease: (a) Cushings syndrome (b) aldosteronism (c) phaeochromocytoma
iii. Systemic disorders: (a) systemic lupus erythematosus (b) poly-arteritis nodosa (c) scleroderma (d) toxaemia of pregnancy.
iv. Coarctation of the aorta
v. Intracerebral lesions
vi. Acute porphyria.

Aetiological factors and mechanism

Blood pressure is normally regulated by two mechanisms: one is mediated by the nervous system with afferent and efferent pathways in the sympathetic system acting through a reflex arc involving the brain stem which is also influenced by impulses from the cerebral cortex; the other system is a humoral one depending on the kidneys and adrenal glands and the renin-angiotensin-aldosterone system.

The neurogenic mechanism

Vasoconstriction is mediated by the beta-adrenergic nerves but there is no evidence that excessive production of catecholamines which would stimulate them is the primary cause of high blood pressure. A normal level of pressure is maintained by reflex arcs derived from stretch receptors in the arteries and in the carotid sinus and although the level of homeostasis is set abnormally high with sustained high blood pressure, there is no evidence that this is the primary cause of the condition. Abnormal efferent stimuli from the cerebral cortex due to emotion or anxiety can raise the blood pressure but there is no evidence that this mechanism can produce a sustained high level of pressure. The possibility cannot be ruled out that the combination of minor variations in these mechanisms together with an abnormal responsiveness of the arterioles may contribute to the development of persistent high blood pressure.

The humoral mechanism

A proteolytic enzyme *renin* is produced in the kidney by cells near the point where the blood vessels enter the glomerulus— the juxta-glomerular apparatus. The main stimulus to renin production appears to be a reduced effective blood volume 'sensed' as a reduced pressure. Renin converts the plasma protein angiotensinogen to a physiologically inactive polypeptide Angiotensin 1 and this is further changed in the lung to Angiotensin 2. This substance is a powerful vasoconstrictor and it also stimulates the suprarenal glands to an increased production of aldosterone. The latter causes sodium and water retention increasing the plasma volume and therefore raising the blood pressure. The increased output of aldosterone reduces the production of renin so that there is a familiar negative-feed back mechanism, tending to maintain a steady effective blood volume and blood pressure.

This humoral mode of control of the blood pressure appears to be relevant in ischaemic disease of the kidney. Renal artery stenosis or narrowing of the smaller vessels may lower the pressure in the juxta-glomerular apparatus leading to the increased output of renin and activating the angiotensin-aldosterone mechanism. Experimentally the removal of an ischaemic kidney, provided the contralateral kidney is healthy, can reduce a raised blood pressure to normal but in man it does not always do so possibly because secondary changes occur in the opposite kidney before the operation can be performed.

If hypertension persists the renin output and blood levels may gradually fall towards normal probably as a result of the negative-feed back mechanism. In general they remain higher when high blood pressure is due to demonstrable renal disease than in cases in whom there is no discoverable cause and in the latter there is no evidence at present that an abnormality of this humoral mechanism is the initiating cause of the high blood pressure. The kidneys also produce substances which lower the blood pressure as a primary action and renal disease may interfere with this mechanism, but here too there is no evidence in the majority of cases that this is the responsible initiating factor.

As in the neurogenic mechanism it is possible that minor abnormalities at various points in the chain of reactions or abnormalities of sensitivity of the end-organ may combine to produce an abnormal pressure.

Heredity

Heredity is unquestionably a powerful factor in the aetiology of high blood pressure. About 30 per cent of subjects with one hypertensive parent and 45 per cent of those in whom both parents are hypertensive, also suffer from the disorder. If neither parent is hypertensive a raised blood pressure is usually found to be due to a renal or other discoverable cause. The mode of inheritance is disputed. It has been suggested that it is transmitted as a mendelian dominant with a high rate of expression. If this were so the distribution curve of the blood pressure in the population would be bi-modal, the first peak of distribution would show the commonest pressure among normal subjects and the second peak the commonest pressure of subjects with inherited high blood pressure. However, if there are numerous inherited factors and also other environmental factors there would be a uni-modal distribution curve. The type of curve obtained in population studies, however, depends greatly on the selection of subjects examined but although not finally settled, it seems probable that there are many inherited factors and also some environmental factors involved.

In clinical practice a very high blood pressure in a young person with normotensive parents strongly suggests the presence of a discoverable cause. By contrast, the presence of a raised pressure in the parents or siblings makes the hereditary type of raised pressure the probable diagnosis, but it does not exclude the possiblity of a discoverable cause which should be sought if there are other suspicious features.

Pathology

In the absence of an underlying cause the morbid anatomical features are all secondary to the raised blood pressure. There is medial hypertrophy of the arterioles with intimal thickening and concentric hypertrophy of the left ventricle. In the later stages there is also dilatation of the left ventricle and as the blood pressure rises in the left atrium and pulmonary veins there is consequent pulmonary hypertension and hypertrophy of the right heart. The kidneys show coarse scarring due to ischaemia consequent on intimal thickening and atheromatous lesions of the arteries. The kidneys may be considerably shrunken.

Clinical features

Very many subjects have no symptoms directly referable to their raised pressure. Some complain of dizziness and poor mental concentration. Headaches are only attributable to high blood pressure if they are present on waking in the morning, lessen in severity during the day and are prevented by sleeping in a semi-recumbent position. About 5–10 per cent of cases have angina of effort. As the disease develops there may be effort dyspnoea or the dramatic development of paroxysmal nocturnal dyspnoea due to pulmonary oedema. Finally congestive heart failure may occur and sometimes this happens without evidence of preceding left ventricular failure. In congestive heart failure the blood pressure occasionally rises, but often remains the same and sometimes falls. In the latter case the cause of the heart failure may be difficult to determine if the previous blood pressure is unknown and if the ocular fundi do not show abnormalities.

At first the only physical sign is a presystolic heart sound, but later left ventricular hypertrophy may be diagnosed from the character of the cardiac impulse. The ocular fundi show narrowing of the arteries and the veins are nipped where the arteries cross them. In more advanced cases there may be small discrete exudates with sharply defined margins occurring particularly in the macular region and sometimes accompanied by flame-shaped haemorrhages. Ill-defined 'cotton-wool' exudates suggest the imminence of the accelerated phase and papilloedema is diagnostic of it (see later in this chapter).

As the disease develops the presystolic heart sound gives place to a third heart sound and if there is a tachycardia a gallop cadence is produced. Pulsus alternans may occur when there is left ventricular failure. Atrial fibrillation, which may be paroxysmal, develops in about 7 per cent of cases. If there is congestive failure, a raised venous pressure, hepatic enlargement and oedema are added to the above signs.

Clinical features of the accelerated phase

The accelerated phase is a rare condition, often presenting

abruptly in patients below the age of 40 years. It may result from any of the known causes of a high blood pressure, and may also terminate a long course of high blood pressure of unknown cause. It affects men as often as women, in contrast to the usual sex incidence of high blood pressure. Symptoms are abrupt and depend upon the organs dominantly involved by the arterial lesion. If these are cerebral there may be morning headaches, loss of mental concentration with intellectual impairment, drowsiness, convulsions and coma. There may be transient or permanent paralyses or amblyopia (hypertensive encephalopathy). Loss of visual acuity may be caused by extensive ill-defined 'cotton-wool' exudates and haemorrhages in the fundi and papilloedema is diagnostic of the condition. The urine contains albumen, hyaline and granular casts, and red cells. The diastolic blood pressure is usually above 120 mmHg and often above 140 mmHg, but there may be relatively little left ventricular hypertrophy unless the blood pressure has been raised for a long time. A fourth heart sound is usually audible and the patient may present with nocturnal or effort dyspnoea.

Signs of any of the primary causes of hypertension may be present with the sole exception of aortic coarctation. In this condition, the accelerated phase does not occur presumably because the renal arterioles are protected by the aortic constriction from the excessively high pressure which produces the necrotising arteriolar lesion.

The blood urea is usually raised and there may be a mild hypokalaemic alkalosis due to secondary aldosteronism. In contrast to primary aldosteronism due to an adenoma, patients with malignant hypertension rarely have a serum potassium below 3mEq/l and the serum sodium is often reduced as well.

The prognosis is very bad and nearly all untreated patients die within two years. Immediate treatment with hypotensive drugs is one of the few medical emergencies and good control of the blood pressure can prolong life for 5 to 10 years in many patients.

The cardiogram

This may be normal in mild and early cases. Later there may be signs of left ventricular hypertrophy at first with increased voltage only; one or more of the limb leads exceeds 15 mm in height or the sum of S in V1 and R in V5 or 6 exceeds 35 mm. Later there may be T wave inversion in lead 1 and V5 or 6 and this is an ominous sign. Broadening and notching of the P wave in lead 1 provides further evidence of left heart enlargement by showing left atrial enlargement.

Radiology

This is less sensitive than the cardiogram in showing left ventricular enlargement since it depends on dilatation as well as hypertrophy before the left ventricular enlargement is apparent. In the late stages pulmonary oedema may be visible as fan-shaped opacities radiating from the hilar regions.

The urine

This usually contains no more than a faint trace of albumen with a few hyaline casts.

Biochemical investigations

Several biochemical investigations are of importance because they may point to an underlying cause and assist both prognosis and treatment. The serum cholesterol and triglycerides and fasting glucose are important prognostic factors. A slightly raised serum creatinine or blood urea indicates renal involvement which may be primary or due to the high blood pressure, but considerably raised levels suggest a primary renal cause of the high pressure. The uric acid is often elevated even when there is no overt gout and points to the need for caution in treatment with diuretics. A high serum sodium with low potassium associated with considerable potassium excretion in the urine in the absence of diuretic therapy suggests the presence of an adenoma of the suprarenals (Conn's syndrome) and suggests the need for further confirmatory tests such as estimation of the plasma renin if this is feasible or a therapeutic test using the aldo-sterone antogonist, Aldactone, to try to reverse the clinical features and electrolyte pattern. A screening test for phaeo-chromocytoma by looking for catecholamine derivatives in the urine, such as vanillomandelic acid (VMA), is now very simple and can be applied to all patients. It is important that hypotensive therapy and broad spectrum antibiotics and phenothiazines are withheld before the tests. If it is positive or if suspicion of the diagnosis is very strong further investigation is best undertaken in a specialized centre (p. 142).

Intravenous pyelography

Almost all patients with high blood pressure should have an intravenous pyelogram performed. Exceptions may be made in the elderly or sometimes in those who have at least two siblings with high blood pressure, but of course it must not be forgotten that the presence of such a family history does not exclude the possibility of an underlying remediable cause. The pyelogram may show any of the renal causes of hypertension listed above. Delayed and concentrated excretion of the contrast on one side suggests the possibility of renal artery stenosis and indicates the need for an aortogram with selective visualisation of the renal arteries and also perhaps divided renal function studies by ureteric catheterisation. Such studies may also be demanded by the finding of a unilateral shrunken kidney but will usually only be possible in specialised units.

Prognosis

It has been shown that mortality is closely related to the height both of the systolic and diastolic blood pressure. It rises smoothly from levels of 110/75 to over 280/120 with no abrupt change at any point and for men the mortality at the higher value is 2.8 times that at the lower value. Clearly high blood pressure can be injurious to health but in the individual case a patient can live for very many years with it. It has been possible to identify a number of factors which conduce to a bad prognosis. Many of them do so by predisposing to coronary artery disease or to cerebro-vascular disease. They include the height of the systolic or diastolic blood pressure, cigarette smoking, glucose intolerance, left ventricular hypertrophy in the cardiogram, a raised serum cholesterol or triglycerides, obesity and albuminuria. These adverse features are additive—the more there are, the worse the prognosis. At one end of the spectrum of high blood pressure there is the patient with simply a raised pressure and no other features with a prognosis which may be uneventful for 10 or 15 years, and at the other end a patient with cardiographic evidence of left ventricular hypertrophy and albuminuria in whom the prognosis may be as short as 2 years. Between these extremes there are various gradations according to the presence of the other adverse factors mentioned. These subjects are at risk from angina, cardiac infarction, congestive failure or cerebro-vascular accidents.

Treatment

General measures

Work and emotional stress raise the blood pressure while relaxation and sleep lower it. The patient's personal habits must therefore be carefully reviewed. He must avoid unecessary or excessive business or social commitments and nine hours rest in bed must be obtained every night. Diazepam (Valium) 2 mg twice or thrice daily may be given to reduce emotional tension by day and secure sufficient sleep at night. Weight must be reduced to the optimum level but alcohol in strict moderation may be allowed. Smoking must be absolutely forbidden.

Indications for the use of drugs

It has been shown that the prognosis is greatly improved if the blood pressure can be maintained below 150/90 mmHg and ideally all patients whose pressures persistently exceed this level should be treated with drugs. Since the risk of development of complications begins at an even lower level it has been argued that all patients whose pressure exceeds 140/90 mmHg should be treated similarly. However, there are many difficulties in pursuing this ideal including the cost, the numbers of patients involved and the difficulty of persuading asymptomatic subjects to accept the prospect of life-long medication for what must be admitted to be a conjectural benefit in the individual case. The decision to treat a patient with a slightly raised pressure is therefore based on the number of adverse features he shows. These include a family history of high blood pressure, incorrigible cigarette smoking, glucose intolerance and hyperlipidaemia. Naturally all patients with cerebral, renal or cardiac involvement will require drug treatment.

Although many powerful drugs are now available for reduction of the blood pressure none is entirely satisfactory or completely without undesirable side effects. For this reason all but the mildest cases will require a combination of two or more drugs so that the dose of each is kept relatively low and its side-effects minimised. Nevertheless many patients do not feel as well on treatment as without it. A compromise has sometimes to be made between an optimal reduction of the pressure and one that is tolerable to the patient, but in serious cases the patient may have to be strongly encouraged to put up with unpleasant side effects.

The drugs are first described separately and then suggestions are made for their use in combination:

1. *Diuretics*
   a. Bendrofluazide 5 mg on alternate days or daily
   b. Chlorthalidone (Hygroton) 50–100 mg daily
This has a gradual and prolonged action lasting for about twenty-four hours.

These substances have a mild or moderate hypotensive effect but greatly potentiate the action of the stronger drugs listed below. They are relatively free of side effects but acute gout may be precipitated in patients with a raised serum uric acid level. This can be prevented by giving Allopurinol 100 mg three times a day. Other side effects of diuretics are uncommon but may include dyspepsia, allergic reaction, rashes and muscular weakness.

2. *Drugs which reduce the peripheral resistance by an action on the central nervous system*
   a. Methyl Dopa (Aldomet) 0.5–2.0 g/day in divided doses.
This is the most generally useful drug in the group as it is moderately powerful and rarely loses its effectiveness. Side effects are uncommon but may include drowsiness, which is usually transient, dyspepsia, oedema and haemolytic anaemia. A positive Coombe's test without anaemia often occurs and treatment can be continued in spite of it.

b. Clonidine (Catapres) 0.1–0.3 mg three times daily. This is a moderately powerful drug which may cause some sedation.

3. *Drugs blocking beta-receptors*
   a. Propranolol (Inderal) 40–180 mg three times daily.
   b. Oxprenolol (Trasicor) 80–160 mg three times daily.
These drugs block B-adrenergic receptors of the heart reducing the force and frequency of contraction. They may therefore prevent sudden increases of cardiac output and condition the baroceptors to maintain a permanently lower level of pressure. They may also diminish aldosterone production and thus reduce water and salt retention. They are relatively free of side effects and do not produce postural hypotension but must be avoided in asthmatics and patients with actual or incipient heart failure.

4. *Drugs acting on adrenergic nerve endings*
   a. Bethanidine (Esbatal) 10–300 mg twice daily.
   b. Guanethidine (Ismelin) 10–80 mg once daily.
These are powerful drugs with unpleasant side effects which include muscular weakness, dizziness, postural hypotension, fluid retention, failure of ejaculation and impotence.

5. *Peripheral vasoldilators*
   a. Prazosin (Hypovase) 1–6 mg three times daily.
Prazosin causes arteriolar dilatation by direct action on the smooth muscle of the blood vessels. Occasionally the first dose produces an exaggerated response with a profound fall of pressure and fainting on standing. It should therefore be given after food at night and the patient is told to remain in bed after taking the tablet. The reaction rarely follows subsequent doses. Other adverse reactions seem to be uncommon but may include drowsiness, lethargy, dry mouth, depression and bowel disturbances.

The use of drugs in combination
In all but the severest cases a start should be made with the mildest drugs which give the fewest side effects and more potent drugs are added only if an adequate reduction of pressure is not obtained.

In most cases a thiazide diuretic is the drug of first choice and then Methyl Dopa or Propranolol is added if necessary. The latter is particularly appropriate if the patient also has angina but is contra-indicated if there is imminent or actual heart failure. If control is not achieved with this combination both Propranolol and Methyl Dopa can be given together with the diuretic or Bethanidine or Clonidine is added.

The treatment of severe or accelerated hypertension or hypertensive encephalopathy is a medical emergency and the blood pressure must be promptly reduced by parenteral therapy. Diazoxide in a dose of 300 mg in an intravenous bolus is probably the drug of first choice. Alternatively Clonidine in a dose of 500 mg in 500 ml of 5 per cent Dextrose, or Methyl Dopa 50–100 mg, or Reserpine 1–2.5 mg i.m. or Guanethidine 10–20 mg i.m. 4-hourly can be used. Parenteral dosage is gradually reduced as oral administration is substituted.

It must be emphasized that the hypertensive regime must be individually designed in each case according to the patient's needs and the side effects produced. There is a wide variation in the occurrence of unwanted effects and in the doses needed to produce adequate responses. Sometimes trial has to be made of many different combinations of drugs before one is found which produces adequate control with a minimum of unpleasant symptoms. Finally it must be understood both by the patient and the doctor that treatment once instituted is likely to be required for the remainder of the patient's life, and that regular measurements of the blood pressure must be made in the recumbent, sitting and standing positions, aiming to maintain a systolic pressure in young patients below 145 mmHg and a diastolic pressure below 90 mmHg. In older patients a systolic pressure below 160 mmHg and diastolic pressure below 95 mmHg may have to be accepted. Once a satisfactory pressure is achieved the dosage should not be altered unless an unexpected fall of pressure occurs during an infection or for some other unexpected reason.

FURTHER READING

Hypertension (1976) Symposium *American Journal of Medicine*, **60**, 733–903.
Kannel, W.B. (1974) Role of blood pressure in cardiovascular morbidity and mortality. *Progress in Cardiovascular Disease*, **17**, 5.
Pickering, G., (1974) *Hypertension*. London: J & A Churchill.

10. Phaeochromocytoma

Pathology

Phaeochromocytoma is a tumour of chromaffin tissue and characteristically occurs in a suprarenal gland. Occasionally, however, it may be found elsewhere, especially in the neighbourhood of the sympathetic chain, behind the inferior vena cava, in the wall of the bladder or even in the chest. Occasionally the tumours are multiple and in a small proportion of cases they are malignant. The tumour secretes adrenalin and noradrenalin, resulting in a striking clinical picture.

Clinical features

The tumour may produce either paroxysmal or sustained arterial hypertension but only 0.5 per cent of cases of hypertension are caused by a phaeochromocytoma. If it causes paroxysmal hypertension there may be sudden attacks of violent headache, nocturnal dyspnoea or pulmonary oedema or angina. The attacks may be accompanied by apprehension, sweating, trembling and palpitations. During the attacks the patient is usually pale but afterwards he may be flushed and there may be swelling of the thyroid gland, the cause of which is uncertain. In cases with sustained hypertension there is excessive sweating, a raised metabolic rate with weight loss, and a marked hypertensive retinopathy. Unless one of these three features is present a phaeochromocytoma need not be seriously considered as the cause of sustained hypertension. The excessive production of adrenalin may result in glycosuria and there is often albumenuria as well.

Diagnosis

The most reliable method of establishing the diagnosis is by estimation of the urinary catecholamines, which are normally present in a concentration of less than 12 μg per litre. If there is an actively secreting tumour the value may reach several hundred or even thousands of micrograms. It is easier, however, to estimate or examine the urine qualitatively for Vanyl-Mandelic acid (V.M.A.), a breakdown product of catecholamines.

Adrenalin and noradrenalin are specifically antagonised by Rogitine and if a dose of 5 mg intravenously produces a fall of blood pressure exceeding 35 mmHg systolic and 25 mmHg diastolic it strongly suggests the presence of a phaeochromocytoma. Further investigations are complicated. Radiological visualisation of the tumour may be attempted by combining intravenous pyelography with peri-renal or pre-sacral carbon-dioxide insufflation. The catecholamine content of adrenal vein and inferior vena caval blood may be estimated by retrograde catheterisation via the femoral vein. These examinations are best made in specialized centres.

Differential diagnosis

In paroxysmal cases the differentiation of an anxiety state which may produce sweating, palpitations, trembling, a raised metabolic rate and hypertension may be extremely difficult and depends upon the discovery of an adequate cause for the neurosis and the repeated absence of excess catecholamines or V.M.A. from the urine. Hyperthyroidism can be distinguished by radio-iodine uptake studies. Attacks closely resembling those caused by a phaeochromocytoma may occur in the menopause but are accompanied by flushes rather than pallor. Other causes of sustained hypertension do not usually cause sweating, trembling or raised metabolic rate with weight loss.

Treatment

The tumour or tumours must be removed and it is important to explore both suprarenals. If the tumour is not found there, the renal pelvis and the region of the entire sympathetic chain must be examined. The blood pressure may need to be controlled with Rogitine before operation and during it with Phenoxybenzamine, and Propranolol as a dangerous rise of pressure may occur while the tumour is being handled due to liberation of adrenalin and noradrenalin. As the venous drainage of the tumour is ligated, noradrenalin in a dose of ten micrograms per minute may be needed to maintain a normal pressure.

11. Ischaemic Heart Disease

Definition

Disease of the heart due to obstruction of the coronary arteries by atheroma.

Aetiology

These are several well-known predisposing factors in the aetiology of ischaemic heart disease. There is often a strong hereditary or familial incidence although whether this is truly genetic or merely environmental is uncertain. The disease has its maximum incidence in men between the ages of 45 and 55 years and in women between 55 and 65 years, that is to say about 10 years after the menopause. This difference in peak incidence appears to be related to ovarian function. If the ovaries are removed before the menopause, ischaemic heart disease may be found correspondingly prematurely. But the disease is becoming more common affecting both sexes at progressively earlier ages, though the different sex incidence is maintained. Additional predisposing factors are high blood pressure, obesity and cigarette smoking. It is very doubtful whether the so-called 'stresses' of our present mode of life play a direct part in causation.

Certain occupations, including doctors and other professional classes, executives and sedentary workers, show a relatively high incidence while manual workers and those undertaking other forms of physical activity at work have a lower incidence. Physical activity certainly has some preventive effect but the occupational differences may be partly due to different dietary habits of various social classes. A high intake of animal fat has for long been a suspected aetiological factor. In Germany, during the First World War, when animal fat was scarce, there was a remarkable reduction in the incidence of ischaemic heart disease. A study of three racial groups in South Africa showed correlations between the incidence of coronary disease, consumption of animal fat and serum lipids.

Hyperlipidaemia

Lipids are substances soluble in ether-alcohol and the important ones in ischaemic heart disease are cholesterol and triglycerides. These circulate in the blood in combination with protein (lipoproteins) in particles of various sizes in which the proportion of cholesterol to triglycerides differs (Fig. 11.1).

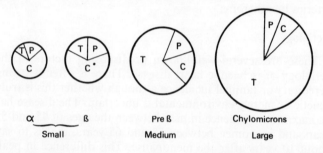

Fig. 11.1 The composition and nomenclature of lipoprotein particles separable by electrophoresis. T = Triglycerides; P = Phospholipids; C = Cholesterol. The encircling black band represents protein. The *small* alpha and beta particles (S—Stone and Thorp) contain a high proportion of cholesterol. If they are considerably increased in number the serum cholesterol is raised but the triglycerides may be normal. The *M*edium-sized pre-beta particles (M—Stone and Thorp) and *L*arge chylomicrons (L—Stone and Thorp) contain a high proportion of triglycerides. An increase in their number raises the serum triglycerides but the serum cholesterol may be normal.

The serum cholesterol and triglycerides can be estimated chemically and the proportions of the different sized particles can be estimated by electrophoresis or by nephelometry. The latter is a simple method depending on the light-scattering power of particles suspended in a fluid. The amount of light-scatter depends on particle size and the proportion of different size particles can be calculated.

The hyperlipidaemias can be classified on the basis of these investigations. The most widely used classification is that of Fredrickson based on chemical estimations and electrophoresis. It can be easily related to the classification of Stone and Thorp based on nephelemetry. The classifications, data on which they are based, and clinical correlations are summarized in Figures 11.1 and 11.2.

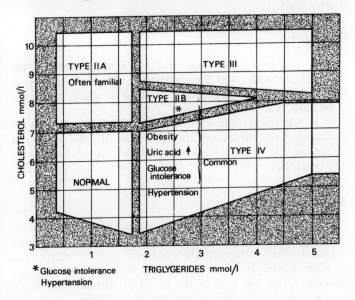

Fig. 11.2 Classification of hyperlipidaemia according to cholesterol and triglyceride levels (Fredrickson).

Types IIa and IIb and Type IV account for the vast majority of hyperlipidaemias and are the most relevant to coronary disease.

Treatment of hyperlipidaemias. It is still uncertain whether reduction and maintenance of lipids at or near normal levels reduces the risk of clinical manifestations of coronary disease.

1. *Diet*

The serum lipids can often be reduced by 20 per cent by the following dietary modifications:

　　a. Fish or poultry is substituted for all but three meat meals per week.

　　b. Margarine is substituted for butter.

c. Vegetable oil is used for cooking.

d. Dairy produce is restricted. Cream and whole milk are not taken but skimmed milk may be used. Eggs are limited to 3 or 4 per week and cheese, except 'cottage cheese', is strictly limited.

Type IIb and Type IV are also helped by carbohydrate restriction.

2. *Drugs*

a. Clofibrate (Atromid–S) 1.5–2 G/daily reduces the serum triglycerides and the cholesterol to a lesser extent. It potentiates oral anticoagulants the dose of which may have to be reduced.

b. Cholestyramine (Questran) 16–32 G/day acts as an exchange resin increasing the excretion of bile acids and cholesterol. It is unpleasant to take and may cause nausea and diarrhoea.

Morbid anatomy

The essential lesion consists of nodular thickenings in the main branches of the coronary system by masses of lipoid material which interrupt the continuity of the elastic and collagen fibres. It is not certain whether these lesions first develop within the wall of the vessel or whether they begin as platelet thrombi within the lumen and later acquire an intimal covering and cholesterol deposits, though the latter seems more probable. The lesions partially occlude the lumen of the vessel and complete occlusion may occur either by the deposition of a further platelet thrombus or occasionally by haemorrhage into the atheromatous lesion. Quite often the anterior descending branch of the left coronary artery is severely affected at a single point 2 cm from its origin while the remaining vessels are relatively healthy, but in the majority of cases there is widespread involvement of both right and left coronary vessels and their main branches.

Myocardial infarction may result from occlusion of a major vessel but sometimes occurs in its absence, though in such cases, there is always serious disease of at least two major vessels. The precise mechanism of infarction in such cases is not clear. It has even been suggested that the infarction results simply from increased oxygen demands of the muscle in the presence of a restricted coronary flow and that thrombotic occlusion, when it is found, is the result and not the cause of the infarction. In other cases thrombotic occlusion is found in the absence of infarction. This is presumably explained by the presence of an adequate collateral circulation. The infarct is at first red owing to extravasation of the red cells (infarct means 'stuffed in' with red cells) and later becomes white as the necrotic muscle swells and squeezes out the extravasated blood. Finally the necrotic mass is replaced by fibrous tissue. In some cases in which the full thickness of the muscle is involved and finally replaced by fibrous tissue, this may form an area which balloons out under the force of the intraventricular pressure forming an aneurysm. This may have serious haemodynamic consequences since part of the output of the left ventricle is diverted into the sac. The systemic circulation is robbed of this volume and the situation is comparable to that of mitral reflux in which part of the left ventricular output is diverted into the left atrium. As a result left ventricular failure may occur with its attendant symptoms.

Infarction may occur in the antero-septal region (where it occasionally results in perforation of the septum), anterolaterally, laterally, inferiorly (formerly called posterior), or infero-laterally. An infarction in either of the last two sites may involve the papillary muscles of the mitral valve and cause mitral reflux.

Haemodynamics

Narrowing of the coronary arteries by atheroma upsets the normal self-regulating mechanism which adjusts coronary blood flow, and therefore oxygen supply, to myocardial needs. As the coronary arteries are the first branches of the aorta they are the first to receive any increment of blood resulting from an increased cardiac output. Moreover a rise of blood pressure whether produced by emotion, stooping, exercise or vasoconstriction from cold, also increases coronary flow by raising the filling pressure. If therefore, heart work is increased by a raised output or by a raised arterial pressure, increased coronary flow can and should occur immediately. If the coronary arteries are narrowed, these self-adjusting mechanisms are impeded or prevented, and injury to the myocardium results. This may be transient and reversible if the disproportion between coronary flow and heart work is relatively brief as in exercise, exposure to cold, emotion or hypertension; it is then accompanied by pain but is objectively demonstrable only by temporary depression of the ST segment of the cardiogram. However, if there is a long-lasting disproportion between work and coronary flow, cardiac infarction results. This may occur without complete occlusion of a vessel if there is a very severe reduction of flow with a poor collateral supply, and conversely a complete coronary occlusion does not cause infarction if there is an adequate collateral circulation.

It may be noted, *en passant*, that narrowing of the coronary arteries is only one of several mechanisms which can adversely affect the relationship between heart work and oxygen supply. Other conditions which may increase heart work and diminish coronary flow sufficiently to cause angina include, aortic and pulmonary valve stenosis and pulmonary hypertension (p. 211) Reduction of the mean aortic pressure in aortic reflux also diminishes coronary flow and though anaemia diminishes the oxygen carrying capacity of the blood, angina does not occur unless the anaemia is severe and there is some coronary disease as well.

Clinical presentation

Since coronary occlusion can be recognised clinically only by its effects in producing pain or infarction, and because occlusion and infarction can occur independently of one another, the term coronary thrombosis should be avoided and the following terms used to describe the clinical varieties of ischaemic heart disease:

1. *Angina pectoris* (literally a 'choking of the chest').

A pain with certain characteristic features which may be accompanied by cardiographic signs. There are two varieties:

    a. *Angina of effort*

    b. *Episodic and linked angina*

2. *Cardiac infarction*

A morbid anatomical lesion with characteristic clinical, cardiographic and biochemical features.

Angina pectoris (Angina of effort)

Clinical features. The recognition of *angina pectoris* depends almost entirely upon the history and special care must be taken to ensure that the patient is using words in the same sense as the physician. The skilled use and interpretation of leading questions is indispensable. If doubt remains when the history is complete it may be necessary to reiterate certain points phrasing the questions differently. The whole procedure may take thirty minutes or more and is one of the most fascinating investigations in clinical practice. (Wood 1969) The pain of angina of effort has four characteristic features:

1. *The site of the pain.* The pain is felt in the midline anywhere from the throat to the xiphisternum and may spread thence to either side of the front of the chest. It may also radiate to the throat, lower jaw, the inner or outer border of one or both arms as far as the fingers, or to the interscapular region (Fig. 11.3). Occasionally it occurs in one or other of these sites of radiation in the absence of pain in the chest. It is rarely confined to the left inframammary region and this site is strongly against the diagnosis.

2. *The quality of the pain.* Angina is a steady, continuous pain with a characteristic choking quality and is often accompanied by belching. It may also be described as tight, bursting, squeezing, 'like a weight', or burning, or simply as 'indescribable'. The patient may also say that he 'cannot get his breath' but enquiry reveals that there is no tachypnoea but merely a sense of constriction or oppression in the chest. Although the pain may be said to be 'sharp' it is rarely stabbing and never shooting or pricking. Its severity ranges from very slight to unbearable and this does not assist diagnosis. The patient often places his clenched fist over the upper sternum as he describes his symptoms, and this is a characteristic and valuable sign.

Many patients and nearly all doctors suffering from angina attribute their pain and discomfort to '*indigestion*' and this symptom should be deliberately sought and carefully analysed whenever it is mentioned; it will often be found to have all the features of angina.

3. *The relationship of pain to increased heart work.* As its name implies the onset of angina of effort is always related

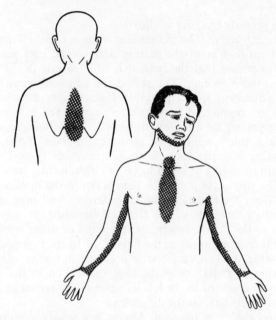

Fig. 11.3 The distribution of ischaemic cardiac pain. The characteristic sites and radiation are shown by the hatched areas.

to an increase in heart work though this may not necessarily be due to *physical* effort. Emotion, food or exposure to cold all have the same effect. It must also be specially emphasized that recumbency and stooping or squatting all produce a dramatic rise of cardiac output and systemic blood pressure through increased venous return, and any of these movements can therefore cause angina.

The amount of effort required to produce pain cannot be expected to be constant as there are so many contributory factors. A walk of 100 yards on a cold day after a meal may provoke pain while the same patient without food on a warm day may be able to walk one mile without pain.

4. *The duration of the pain*. The patient usually learns to stop the effort which led to the pain and *stands still*. The pain disappears in a matter of minutes; if it takes longer than a

quarter of an hour the diagnosis may be episodic angina, cardiac infarction or non-cardiac pain. However, it must be remembered that pain makes time seem to pass slowly and the patient may over-estimate the duration. Cross-questioning will clarify this.

The patient must always be asked specifically whether there has at any time been an attack lasting longer than 15 minutes, perhaps occurring at rest, or in the night and attributed to 'indigestion'. Such an attack may have been due to coronary occlusion without clinical infarction. Prolonged attacks can also be provoked by paroxysmal tachycardia and the patient should always be asked whether they were accompanied by palpitations.

Physical signs. Often there are no abnormal physical signs but it is important to exclude predisposing factors including sub-thyroidism, chronic nephritis, diabetes, hypertension, premature menopause or medication with the contraceptive 'pill'. If the history has made it clear that the patient has angina, the cause may be coronary atheroma, or some other form of heart disease, including aortic valve disease, pulmonary stenosis or extreme pulmonary hypertension as previously mentioned. Anaemia may be a contributory factor.

The fourth heart sound is sometimes audible especially if pain is present and unless otherwise explicable strongly supports the diagnosis. Generalized occlusive vascular disease should be sought be palpating all the peripheral pulses and listening over the iliac and femoral arteries for murmurs due to partial obstruction. Predisposing diseases including diabetes, gout, sub-thyroidism, and hypertension should be sought.

The cardiogram. This is normal unless another form of heart disease is present or there has been a previous infarction or the patient is suffering the pain at the time the record is made. In the latter case the ST segment is horizontal and depressed or slopes downwards in leads V4–6, returning to normal after the pain disappears. In difficult cases it may be necessary to perform an effort test to determine whether the patient's symptoms are accompanied by these characteristic changes. The test carries a very small but definite risk of provoking cardiac infarction or even sudden death but if certain precautions are scrupulously observed, it can be used with confidence when the diagnosis is in doubt. These precautions are as follows:

1. The test should *not* be carried out if the resting cardiogram is abnormal.

2. The test must *not* be performed if the history of supposed angina is of less than four weeks duration,

3. A doctor must supervise the test to decide when it should terminate.

The patient must be exercised until the symptoms of which he complains occur. The cardiogram is then recorded as quickly as possible and further recordings are repeated at intervals for ten minutes or until the record has returned to its resting state. Leads V3–6 usually give all the essential information. The differentiation of ST depression due to ischaemia from that due to the effect of exercise alone is shown in Figure 6.21. The test is positive in over 80 per cent of cases in whom the diagnosis seems likely or certain on clinical grounds and false positives are probably rare provided that the pitfalls illustrated are avoided. In a few cases the test is negative although serious disease is shown angiographically. Another small group of cases show normal angiograms and effort tests although the history is characteristic of angina.

Differential diagnosis:

1. *Left infra-mammary pain associated with an anxiety state.* This is the commonest problem in diagnosis and such pain occurs in two -forms. One is a sudden, severe, stabbing, knife-like pain occurring on effort, below the nipple. It causes the patient to halt abruptly and 'catch his breath', but disappears as quickly as it came. The other is a prolonged aching, stabbing or pricking pain in the same region, unrelated to effort. It must be remembered that these 'anxiety-pains' commonly co-exist with ischaemic cardiac pain because many patients with ischaemic heart disease not unnaturally suffer from an enxiety state.

2. *'Indigestion'.* It has already been noted that patients suffering from angina commonly call their symptom 'indigestion', particularly as it is often worse after food and accompanied by aerophagy and belching. Differentiation, however, is usually easy, for dyspepsia is usually related *only* to food while angina is rarely produced *solely* in this way.

3. *Hiatus hernia.* This is often a difficult differential diagnosis as the pain may be similar in site and quality to that of angina and in both diseases it may be precipitated by recumbency and stooping. Hiatus hernia is a common condition and does not always cause pain so that its presence does not exclude the possibility of angina. However, serious diagnostic difficulty only occurs in patients with nocturnal or episodic pain in whom a cardiogram taken during the attack may be needed to establish the diagnosis.

4. *Cervical spondylosis.* In this condition pain often predominates in the arms but tends to occur *after* effort and to last longer than angina. The discovery of neurological signs in the arms and narrowing of intervertebral foramina in an X-ray of the cervical spine clinches the diagnosis.

Prognosis. The course of angina of effort is one of relapses due to fresh or worsening lesions and partial remissions due perhaps to the development of collateral vessels, but the general trend is usually one of deterioration sometimes punctuated by episodes of infarction. The latter may be heralded by the sudden recurrence or rapid worsening of angina and if this occurs, complete rest and treatment with anticoagulants should be advised. If the patient escapes both infarction and sudden death, the symptom may persist with relapses and remissions for many years.

Treatment. The nature of the disease must be explained to the patient and the possibility of remissions stressed, for the diagnosis carries almost as ominous a connotation to the lay mind as cancer. For this reason circumlocution should be used and the term 'angina' avoided. He should be cautioned to avoid sudden strenuous exertion, particularly after food or in the cold, but allowed to take steady accustomed exercise within the limits imposed by his pain. He should be told to stop when this occurs and wait until it has completely subsided before resuming activity. Relief may be hastened if Tab. Glyceryl Trinitrate 0.5 mg is slowly chewed. The patient must be warned that this will produce flushing and possibly headache but that these effects usually disappear with persistent use. Alternatively Trinitrate may be used before undertaking effort known to produce pain. The drug is not cumulative and 20 tablets or more can be taken each day if necessary.

The only effective long acting nitrates are glyceryl trinitrate 2.6 mg or 6.4 mg in a delayed release tablet (Sustac) and Isosorbide nitrate (Isordil) 10 mg or more thrice daily. Either of these preparations may be useful in patients with repeated attacks. In such cases, however, prevention is usually more effective by the use of beta-adrenergic blockade with propranolol (Inderal). Provided a test dose of 20 mg produces no weakness or faintness 40 mg is given 3 times daily and increased until pain is controlled or until moderate exercise fails to accelerate the heart rate above 80 per minute. This indicates that satisfactory beta-blockade has been achieved and that little will be gained by increasing the dose further. The drug diminishes both the force and frequency of cardiac contraction and surges of output on emotion and exercise are prevented. Side-effects are uncommon but dosage may sometimes have to be modified or the therapy changed if it produces undue bradycardia, depression or lack of energy.

If these measures fail and the patient is disabled by pain a coronary by-pass operation may be advised. A length of the patient's saphenous vein is excised and one end is sutured to the aorta and the other to the coronary artery distal to the block or narrowing. By-passes may be needed on one, two or all three main coronary vessels and preliminary coronary angiography is essential to determine the main sites of obstruction and patency of the vessel beyond.

Episodic and linked angina

In a few patients, attacks of *angina pectoris*, exactly resembling that of angina of effort in site and quality but lacking any connection with an increase of heart work, occur episodically over long or short periods of time. In some cases they may disappear for years or permanently and in others terminate in cardiac infarction. The cardiogram taken after effort may show characteristic ST depression even though no pain was felt at the time.

Treatment of the attack is with nitrates, and if the attacks are frequent prevention may be attempted with beta-blockade.

Finally it should be remembered that patients with angina may also have cervical spondylosis, hiatus hernia, gall-bladder disease or peptic ulceration and the pain of the two conditions may be inextricably linked. The difficulty of separation of the symptoms may be due to several factors including, the closeness of the neurological pathways concerned, the sharing of some features such as relationship to food, and the fact that the pain of these associated diseases provokes anginal attacks.

The demonstration of coronary disease by the cardiogram and the complicating disease by radiology is vital and often rewarding, because successful treatment of the complicating disorder may conspicuously relieve the angina.

Myocardial infarction

Pathology. The pathogenesis and morbid anatomy of coronary atheroma and myocardial infarction have already been discussed. The factors leading to occlusion of the diseased vessel by thrombosis are incompletely understood. Although it has been shown statistically that the coagulability of the blood, and in particular, the adhesiveness of platelets is increased in patients with ischaemic heart disease compared with normal subjects, the frequency of individual exceptions indicates the existence of other unknown factors. Thrombosis is particularly apt to occur when the patient is at rest and the circulation is slowed and also when the coronary circulation is impaired by hypotension due to shock or dehydration. All of these factors are present following surgical operations which themselves cause increased coagulability of the blood.

Haemodynamics. Left ventricular function is impaired to a degree which is usually roughly proportionate to the extent of the infarct. The left ventricular diastolic pressure rises and consequently the left atrial pulmonary venous and pulmonary capillary pressures do so too. The vascular engorgement of the lungs impairs ventilation and gas transport and some fall of arterial oxygen saturation is common. If the pulmonary venous pressure rises considerably pulmonary oedema may occur.

The behaviour of the peripheral arteries is variable. Sometimes there is an initial vaso-vagal reaction with bradycardia and a low blood pressure due to vaso-dilatation. This is usually transient but sometimes there is persistent vaso-dilatation with a low blood pressure and relatively normal cardiac output. In these cases the skin and extremities are warm and tissue and renal perfussion is good. The condition is not dangerous. In other cases there may be vaso-constriction sufficient to produce a rise of blood pressure or at any rate maintenance of a normal level, despite some fall in cardiac output. However, if the latter is considerable the blood pressure falls despite intense vaso-constriction. Reduction of tissue and renal perfusion produces acidosis and oliguria and the condition, which is sometimes called 'cardiogenic shock', is usually fatal.

Clinical features. The attack may occur without previous symptoms or follow a period of worsening angina. It most often occurs when the patient is at rest and may follow unaccustomed physical effort undertaken in the cold. It may strike down an 'after-dinner' speaker through the combined effect of a heavy meal and excitement. The onset is almost invariably marked by characteristic pain identical in site, quality and radiation with that of *angina pectoris* but persistent and uninfluenced by effort. The severity of the pain which ranges from trivial to excruciating, does not help in the diagnosis and is no guide to the severity of the attack. Pain is present in over ninety per cent of cases and if it is absent the diagnosis should be made only if other evidence is very strong. Sometimes the patient denies pain because he attributes the symptom to habitual indigestion or because it is overshadowed by a fainting attack or paroxysmal dyspnoea due to acute left ventricular failure. Only one to two per cent of cases are truly symptomless.

It should be noted that in the majority of cases the apearance of the patient is normal; the blood pressure does not fall, (it may even rise) and there are no abnormal physical signs with the possible exception of an atrial sound. If there is tachycardia the heart sounds may be loud. Exceptionally the onset is marked by a vaso-vagal reaction with bradycardia and hypotension, and in a further few cases there is a fall of blood pressure which may be extreme, together with vaso-constriction producing ashen pallor, a cold clammy skin, restlessness and oliguria or anuria. This condition, called 'cardiogenic shock', is fortunately rare and when it occurs usually fatal. Occasionally the onset is with acute breathlessness due to pulmonary oedema.

During the first few days there is often a low-grade fever

to 37.4°C and in severe attacks it may even rise to 38.4°C for a week or more.

The cardiogram. In normal subjects depolarisation of the left ventricle proceeds from the sub-endocardium outwards during the first 0.04 sec of the QRS interval. The resultant mean vector of these forces usually points inferiorly and to the left in the direction of the long axis of the left ventricle. The necrotic muscle at the centre of an infarction, however, produces no electrical forces and this alters the direction of the mean vector causing it to point *away from* the infarcted area during the first 0.04 sec of the QRS complex. If this initial vector points to the negative pole of a lead it produces an abnormal Q wave 0.04 sec in duration, while if it points to the positive pole it produces an abnormal R wave. Thus the position of the infarct determines the leads which show abnormal Q or R waves (Fig. 11.4).

The T wave vector is also abnormal and like the initial QRS vector it is directed *away from* the infarct; those leads in which it is directed to the negative pole consequently show abnormal inverted T waves as well as abnormal Q waves already described.

It is apparent that in deciding whether a Q wave is abnormal or not the duration of the wave is crucial. It should be measured from the beginning of its downstroke to the point at which it returns to the base line and it is abnormal if it exceeds 0.03 sec. An alternative though less reliable criterion, is the depth of the Q wave, which does not normally exceed one third of the height of the R wave in the same lead. In most cases showing this sign, however, the duration is also abnormal.

Displacement of the S–T segment due to a current of injury from the damaged muscle surrounding the necrotic centre of the infarct may occur and *reciprocal* displacements, with S–T elevation in Leads 1 and the chest leads accompanied by depression in Lead 3, or vice-versa are characteristic (Fig. 11.5).

The evolution of the cardiographic abnormalities. S–T elevation is usually present within the first few hours of a cardiac infarction but Q and T wave abnormalities may be delayed for a day or two or even for a week. The Q waves may be permanent or diminish slowly in width and amplitude over a period of several months. S–T elevation usually persists only for a few hours or days and when present strongly suggest that the infarct is recent; occasionally, however, it persists for months, so that serial cardiograms are always essential

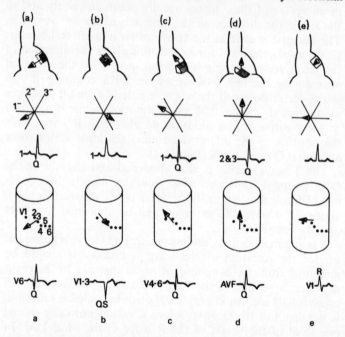

Fig. 11.4 The relation between the position of the infarct, the direction of the 0.04 sec vector and the leads in which abnormal Q or R waves appear. The direction of the 0.04 sec vector is shown pointing away from the site of infarction in five heart diagrams a, b, c, d and e. Below each diagram the vector is redrawn in relation to the axes of the limb leads and below each lead axis diagram is shown the resulting limb lead cardiogram. Below each of these the same vector is drawn within a cylinder on which the chest lead positions are marked, and below each of these the resulting chest lead cardiogram is shown (a, b, c, d, e). (a) The infarct is antero-lateral and abnormal Q waves and inverted T waves appear in leads 1 and V6. (b) The infarct is antero-septal and abnormal QS waves appear in V1–3. (c) The infarct is apical and abnormal Q waves appear in 1, 2 and V4–6. (d) The infarct is inferior ('posterior') and abnormal Q wave appear in 2, 3 and AVF. (e) The infarct is high posterior or lateral and abnormal R waves appear in V1.

to establish the time of the attack with certainty if the clinical picture does not do so. Inversion of the T waves occurs in the first few days, gradually deepening and then lessening over the course of several weeks (Figs. 11.5 and 11.6).

Cardiac infarction without abnormal Q waves. In some cases in which the area of infarction is either small or patchy there is insufficient disturbance of the initial QRS vectors to produce pathological Q waves. Usually however, the T vectors are abnormal and point away from the infarct as already des-

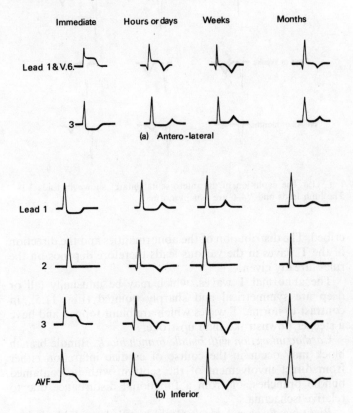

Fig. 11.5 The evolution of the cardiogram in (a) antero-lateral and (b) inferior (posterior) cardiac infarction. In apical infarction the appearances are similar to those in (a) but leads 2 and V4 and 5 may also resemble lead 1.

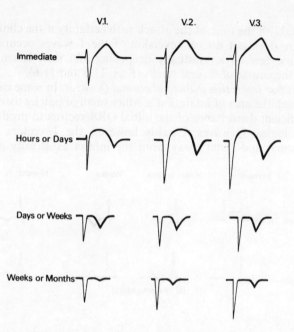

Fig. 11.6 The evolution of an antero-septal infarct shown in leads V1–3. The limb leads and V4–6 are usually normal.

cribed. The distribution of the abnormalities and the direction of the T waves in the various leads therefore depends on the rules already given.

The abnormal T waves, which may be unusually tall or deep are symmetrical and sharply pointed (Fig. 11.5), in contrast to normal T waves which are blunt-topped and have a steeper downstroke than upstroke.

Cardiac infarction with bundle branch block. Bundle branch block may occur in the course of cardiac infarction either from direct involvement of the septum, with its contained bundle branches, or from a functional disturbance due to relative ischaemia.

Right bundle branch block. Right bundle branch block does not alter the initial 0.04 sec. QRS vector, which is produced by the left ventricle. It does not therefore prevent the development of characteristic Q waves. The cardiogram simply shows a combination of the appearances of cardiac infarction with those of bundle branch block (Fig. 11.7).

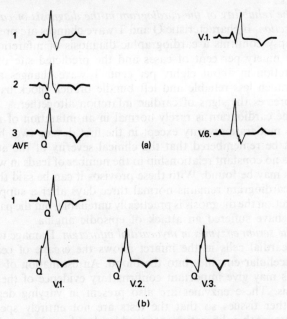

Fig. 11.7(a) Inferior cardiac infarction with right bundle branch block. Bundle branch block is indicated by the broad (0.12 sec) RSR complex in V1 and deep broad S in lead 1 and V6. An inferior infarct is indicated by 0.04 sec Q waves in leads 2 and 3 with inverted T waves. (b) Right bundle branch block is indicated by the wide QRS complex in leads 1 and V1. An antero-lateral infarct is indicated by the broad Q wave in lead 1. An antero-septal infarct is indicated by the presence of Q waves instead of r waves in leads V1–3.

Left bundle branch block. It has been noted (p. 93) that this conduction disturbance produces a characteristic alteration of the initial 0.04 vector which instead of pointing away from the positive poles of Leads 1 and V.4–6 points *toward* them, producing an initial upstroke in these leads and preventing the appearance of normal or abnormal Q waves. Moreover, bundle branch block produces its own S–T depression and T wave inversions in the leads with tall R waves and only if there is T wave inversion in other leads can cardiac infarction be suspected in the presence of left bundle branch block.

The reliability of the cardiogram in the diagnosis of cardiac infarction. If characteristic Q and T wave changes are present, autopsy confirms a cardiographic diagnosis of infarction in over ninety per cent of cases and the predicted site of the infarction in about eighty per cent. T wave changes alone are much less reliable and left bundle branch block usually suppresses the signs of cardiac infarction altogether.

The cardiogram is rarely normal in an infarction of more than moderate severity except in the first day or two, but it must be remembered that the clinical severity of the attack bears no constant relationship to the number of leads in which signs may be found. With these provisos it can be said that if the cardiogram remains normal three days after a supposed infarction the diagnosis is practically untenable, but the patient may have suffered an attack of episodic angina.

The serum enzymes in myocardial infarction. Damage to the myocardial cells in the infarct allows the escape of certain intracellular enzymes into the blood. An estimation of their levels may give important confirmatory evidence of the diagnosis. These enzymes are also present in varying degrees in other tissues so that the tests are not entirely specific. Moreover their liberation into the blood and persistence there, is of relatively short duration and varies with each enzyme. The serum creatine phosphokinase (CPK) is the most specific for heart muscle damage and reaches its peak level at about 24 hours after the infarction and then falls rapidly towards normal which may be reached in 3 to 5 days. This enzyme is present in large quantities in skeletal muscle and damage to that even by intramuscular injections will raise the serum levels. The serum aspartate transferase (formerly SGOT) is much less specific and can be liberated following damage to muscle, brain, liver or pancreas. The serum hydroxybutyric dehydrogenase (HBD) and the serum lactic dehydrogenase (LDH) are related to one another and rise to a maximum at about 3 days and remain elevated longer. They are relatively non-specific and may be elevated in hepatitis, jaundice, drug intoxications, shock and muscle cell damage. Despite these limitations, estimation of all these enzymes is of considerable help in confirming the diagnosis. The time sequence of the blood levels with approximate normal values are shown in Figure 11.8.

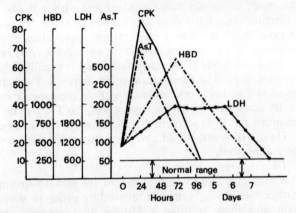

Fig. 11.8 Diagram illustrating the sequential changes in serum enzymes following cardiac infarction. The creatine phosphokinase (CPK) and aspartate transferase (AST) formerly called SGOT, reach a peak in 12–24 hours. The hydroxybutyric dehydrogenase (HBD) and lactic dehydrogenase (LDH) reach their maximum at 72 hours or later.

Differential diagnosis

1. *Massive pulmonary embolism (without pulmonary infarction)*

Differentiation may be very difficult, for the pain of this condition may exactly mimic that of cardiac infarction and may indeed be due to cardiac ischaemia as a result of the low cardiac output. Breathlessness however, is more severe and the venous pressure is often considerably raised. The cardiogram may be diagnostic but sometimes requires 48 hours for its full development. It may show T wave inversion deepest in V1 and lessening towards V4; the T waves become upright successively, first in V4 and then in the other leads, only recovering in V2 and perhaps V1 in four to six weeks. A discoverable source of venous emboli naturally favours the diagnosis. The enzymes, with the exception of CPK, may be considerably raised if there is 'shock' but only the LDH rises in pulmonary infarction without shock.

2. *Pericarditis*

The onset is usually more gradual and although the site and distribution of the pain are similar to those of cardiac infarction, there is often a respiratory aggravation due to involvement of the contiguous pleura. Friction may be heard from the outset while in cardiac infarction it is usually delayed for several days. The cardiogram often shows S–T elevation or inverted T waves in several leads without reciprocal depressions. By contrast with cardiac infarction, the T waves do not invert until the S–T segment has returned to the isoelectric line. The CPK is not raised and the other enzymes are only slightly abnormal.

3. *Diaphragmatic hernia*

This may give rise to pain at rest of the same distribution as cardiac infarction. It may be relieved by sitting or standing upright and there is often a history of numerous similar attacks.

4. *Dissecting aneurysm of the aorta.*

The pain often has a 'tearing' quality and may pass into the abdomen or loins. Abnormal signs in the central nervous system due to involvement of the carotid or intercostal arteries, and asymmetry of the peripheral pulses may be found. The cardiogram may be normal or merely show left ventricular hypertrophy if there was antecedent hypertension, as is commonly the case.

5. *Acute abdominal catastrophes*

Although it is traditionally stressed that acute abdominal catastrophes must always be considered in the differential diagnosis, difficulty does not arise in practice for the pain of cardiac infarction rarely if ever extends below the xiphisternum. Perforation of a peptic ulcer or cholecystitis can usually be differentiated with ease but it must be remembered that a history of 'indigestion' is often given by patients with ischaemic heart disease and belching is common both in cardiac infarction and abdominal conditions. Pancreatitis and cholecystitis occasionally cause some difficulty as they may be accompanied by abnormalities of the T waves but the CPK is not raised and the other enzymes are only slightly affected.

Complications:

1. *Ventricular fibrillation and cardiac standstill*

In the former condition the myocardium shows only fibrillary twitchings and does not contract effectively. These two events are the usual cause of sudden death which is particularly apt to occur during the first two hours following an infarction. Their frequency remains high for 48 hours and gradually diminishes to about the 10th day after which they are relatively rare.

2. *Myocardial rupture*

Perforation of the infarct may occur seven to ten days after the onset in patients undertaking physical exertion and usually results in a fatal haemopericardium.

3. *Dysrhythmias*

Premature beats are common, and if there are more than 5 per minute and arise from the left ventricle (showing a right branch block pattern) they may herald the development of ventricular tachycardia or fibrillation. Transient atrial fibrillation or supraventricular tachycardia or flutter are sometimes seen.

4. *Heart block*

Temporary heart block may result from transient ischaemia of the A–V node which is mainly supplied by the right coronary artery. It therefore occurs most often in patients with an *inferior* infarct, but nearly always disappears if the patient survives, since the infarction does not involve the node. However, if it causes haemodynamic deterioration (which is not invariable) it increases the mortality to 40–50 per cent unless the patient is paced. If atrioventricular block complicates an anterior infarction it is due to involvement of both bundle branches by an extensive infarct and results in a mortality of 80–90 per cent which is scarcely influenced by pacing.

5. *Heart failure*

Patients who have had previous infarctions or who have suffered from hypertensive heart disease, are particularly liable to heart failure.

Left ventricular failure with intense dyspnoea of pulmonary oedema may be the presenting feature of an infarct but congestive failure usually occurs later.

6. *Phlebo-thrombosis*

This is particularly common if the patient is either too ill to move actively in bed or has been made afraid of doing so. The calf veins are frequently involved but more dangerous emboli come from the femoral or pelvic veins. Clinical detection is difficult. Local tenderness over the femoral vein is an important sign but discomfort in the calf when the foot is dorsiflexed with the leg raised (Homan's sign) is very unreliable and the more important proximal thromboses usually defy clinical detection. Prevention by active movement of the legs and regular dorsiflexion of the feet is important.

7. *Arterial emboli*

If the infarct involves the full thickness of the myocardium, a thrombus forms on the endocardial surface within the cavity of the left ventricle. Fragments may become dislodged resulting in embolism of the brain, limbs, gut, kidneys or other organs.

8. *Pericarditis*

If the infarct extends to the epicardium a dry pericarditis with friction results.

9. *Rupture of the papillary muscles or intra-ventricular septum*

Rupture of the papillary muscles is most apt to occur with an inferior infarct and produces severe and usually fatal mitral reflux. The murmur is loudest at the *apex and left axilla*. Rupture of the interventricular septum may follow an antero-septal infarction and produces a *parasternal* systolic murmur and thrill. The lesion usually consists of a sinuous channel allowing communication between the two ventricles and a left-to-right shunt. The condition is commonly but not invariably fatal.

10. *Ventricular aneurysm*

If the infarct is extensive and completely replaced by fibrous tissue it may balloon out with each ventricular contraction. This may reduce the effective left ventricular output sufficiently to lead to symptoms of fatigue, breathlessness or even ultimately to heart failure.

Prognosis. It is difficult to obtain a representative series of patients from which the total survival rate can be calculated; patients who die suddenly are examined by a coroner's pathologist while mild cases are treated at home by their practitioners. Probably the immediate mortality is about 10–20 per cent and unfavourable features are shock, dysrhythmias, heart failure, obesity, diabetes and previous hypertension or cardiac infarction. Of those who survive six weeks, 30 per cent make a complete recovery and the majority of these survive 10 years. 50 per cent however, are left with angina and only half of these live 10 years. 20 per cent may have severe angina or heart failure and are unlikely to live for 5 years.

Treatment

The risk of death is greatest in the first 48 hours from the onset due to cardiac arrest or dysrhythmias which are best treated in hospital. All patients seen during this period are therefore immediately transferred without waiting for confirmation of the diagnosis. The mortality progressively declines until by the tenth day it is low. The need for hospital treatment diminishes correspondingly during this interval and will be judged by the apparent severity of the case, the availability of a coronary care unit and the home circumstances. Before the patient is moved, pain must be relieved with Heroin 5–10 mg i.m., Morphine 10–15 mg i.m. or Pethidine 100 mg i.m. followed by Maxolon 10 mg i.v. or other anti-emetic if vomiting occurs. Serious hypotension may be countered with Metaraminol (Aramine) 4 mg i.m. Ideally the patient should be accompanied by a doctor or ambulance staff trained in cardiac resuscitation.

Rest. Hypotensive patients must lie flat until the pressure rises but all others may be nursed sitting propped up in bed or even in a well padded armchair with a footstool. The cardiac output is lower in a sitting than in a recumbent position due to the reduced venous return and breathing is easier. Moderate or severe cases should be forbidden to wash, feed or shave themselves for about 3 to 5 days but these activities should then be allowed unless there has been hypotension, heart failure or serious dysrhythmias. With the same provisos the patient can be allowed to walk about his room on the 10th day and there is no demonstrable benefit in restricting indoor physical activity after 14 days when the patient can be discharged from hospital.

Diet. This should be restricted to fruit juice and a few dry biscuits for 48 hours. Thereafter meals should be small in bulk and easily digestible and cautiously increased to reach normal in 10 days. A reducing diet is often necessary and a low cholesterol diet is advised if the lipids are raised or become so during the succeeding 3 months.

Anticoagulants. Although controversy exists regarding their value, anticoagulants are generally considered efficacious in reducing the risk of mural and venous thrombi developing and are given to all patients admitted to hospital within 48 hours of the onset, with the exception only of the elderly (say over 70 years), or subjects with a history suggestive of peptic ulceration, liver or kidney disease. Their value in patients seen later or treated at home is more debatable. Treatment is with Heparin 15 000 units intravenously at 12 hours intervals for 48 hours together with an immediate dose of Warfarin 30 mg by mouth. The prothombin time is estimated after 36 hours and subsequent doses of Warfarin, usually ranging from 1–5 mg daily, are necessary to maintain the prothombin time at twice the normal value. Continued anticoagulant treatment for one year may give some protection against further infarction but this belief is not universally accepted and many physicians discontinue anticoagulant treatment when the patient is discharged from hospital or is fully ambulant.

Sedation. After analgesics have been discontinued, Diazepam (Valium) 5–10 mg is given 8 hourly for the first few days.

Oxygen. Nearly all patients with moderate or serious infarction have a reduced arterial oxygen saturation and should be given oxygen at 8 l/min through an oxygenaire safety mask for 24 to 48 hours. If the mask is not well tolerated, 'spectacles' with nasal tubes can be used.

Diuretics. Nearly all patients have some pulmonary oedema which is not often clinically detectable. All should therefore be given an immediate dose of Frusemide (Lasix) 40 mg intravenously or by mouth and the need for further doses assessed each day.

Intravenous fluid. It is useful to maintain a continuous intravenous infusion of 500 ml of 5 per cent Glucose which can be increased to 2–4 l/day if the patient does not take fluids by mouth and into which emergency intravenous therapy can be easily given.

Treatment of complications

Sinus bradycardia. This may result from vagal overaction or Morphine but if the blood pressure is maintained and the general condition is good it is benign and requires no treatment. When associated with an inferior infarction, fall of blood pressure or ventricular premature beats, it may be a precursor of atrio-ventricular block or ventricular fibrillation and should be treated with Atropine 0.6 mg parenterally and repeated as necessary to maintain the heart rate above 60 per minute.

Ventricular premature beats. If these exceed 5 per minute and especially if they arise in the left ventricle (shown by a right bundle branch block pattern on the cardiogram) or are multifocal, they are commonly precursors of ventricular tachycardia or fibrillation and suppression should be attempted with Lignocaine 1–2 mg/kg intravenously followed by a slow infusion of 2–3 mg/min in 5 per cent Glucose for 24 to 48 hours. Overdosage may result in mental confusion, fits, coma or cardiac depression.

Ventricular tachycardia. Treatment is with Lignocaine as described and if it does not respond at once D.C. shock of 350 W/sec. is given followed by 50–80 mEq of Sodium bicarbonate and Lignocaine infusion as described above.

Ventricular fibrillation. This requires immediate cardiac resuscitation, D.C. shock and bicarbonate and Lignocaine infusion. If it recurs, acidosis and hypoxia must be corrected and one or two of the following drugs may be cautiously tried, bearing in mind that all depress cardiac function and are potentially dangerous.

1. Practolol 10 mg intravenously or Propranolol 1–5 mg intravenously followed by oral administration together with Digoxin
  or

2. Mexiletine 100–200 mg I–V, then 200–400 mg 8 hrly. orally.
or
3. Disopyramide (Rythmodan) 300–500 mg/day by mouth
or
4. Procainamide (Pronestyl) 250–500 mg 6 hourly by mouth
or
5. Phenytoin 100–250 mg intravenously slowly every 8 or 12 hours followed by 100–300 mg/day by mouth
or
6. Bretylium Tosylate (Darenthin) 100–200 mg 8 hourly.

Atrio-ventricular block. i. With inferior infarction: A–V block is more commonly associated with inferior than with anterior infarction and is due to transient ischaemia of the A–V node and not to involvement of the His bundle or bundle branches. As a result partial heart block with prolonged P–R interval or progressive prolongation in successive cycles followed by a dropped ventricular beat (Wenkebach phenomenon) are often seen and about half of these cases progress to complete A–V block. If this causes haemodynamic deterioration shown by a fall of blood pressure, cold extremities and oliguria the mortality rises to about 40 per cent and a transvenous pacemaker should be inserted immediately. In other cases no specific treatment need be given and normal conduction almost invariably returns within 3 or 4 days and often within 24 hours. By contrast if a pacemaker has been inserted it may require 1–3 weeks before the patient can be weaned from it.

ii. With anterior infarction. In these cases A–V block is due to extensive involvement of the septum with damage to both bundle branches. Most cases will have shown serious circulatory impairment before the development of block which dramatically worsens their condition. The mortality is about 80 per cent and does not seem to be appreciably improved by pacing.

Supra-ventricular tachycardias. If these cause haemodynamic deterioration they should be treated promptly with DC shock. If there is less urgency, Digoxin is the drug of choice and if this does not control the tachycardia, Propranolol can be added.

Cardiogenic shock. There is no satisfactory treatment for this extremely grave complication. Special care should be taken to ensure that the patient is well oxygenated and repeated estimations should be made of the standard Bicarbonate so that any acidosis can be corrected with Sodium Bicarbonate intravenously. The patient must be kept lying flat to safeguard the cerebral circulation. The patient should be digitalised according to the usual regime. An infusion of 200 ml of 5 per cent Glucose can be given in about 20 minutes and the central venous pressure is watched. Provided it does not rise more than 5 cm above the sternal angle the infusion can be repeated until improvement is shown by the warmer extremities and improved urine output. Vaso-pressor agents such as Metaraminol or Noradrenalin have little if any part to play in the treatment of this condition for although they produce a transient rise of blood pressure through intense vaso-constriction, this results in diminished tissue perfusion and consequent aggravation of acidosis which further impairs cardiac function and may precipitate dangerous arrhythmias. Isoprenaline, which increases the force of the heart-beat without causing generalised vaso-constriction, may sometimes be helpful.

Rehabilitation. It is important that the patient should be told from the outset, that not only are his chances of surviving the attack good, but that there is every likelihood of an eventual resumption of full physical activity and a return to his original occupation. This reassurance should be reiterated at every stage during the patient's illness and convalescence. The latter need not be as prolonged as was once thought necessary. It has been found that patients can be allowed to walk about freely indoors from the 14th day, and out of doors one month from the onset. They should then walk progressively longer distances so that about 8 weeks from the onset they are walking 2 or 3 miles per day and are fit to return to work. If their original occupation involves heavy physical exertion, a further period of physical training may be necessary and is only contra-indicated if there has been heart failure or if there is residual cardiac enlargement, angina or gallop rhythm. Unfortunately although it is now possible to re-train patients physically quite early after cardiac infarction, and thus convince them that they have made a complete recovery from an illness which has probably left no obvious impairment of cardiac function, it is often difficult or impossible to persuade their employers of this. In view of the commonness of the condition and the serious consequences of a failure to return to the previous occupation, it is important that every effort be made to change the attitude of employers to this disease.

Chronic ischaemic heart disease

Pathology

In the late stages of ischaemic heart disease there is atheroma usually of all three main coronary arteries with gross narrowings or occlusions. The myocardium frequently shows large scars of previous infarctions with replacement fibrosis of the muscle. A confluent area of fibrosis may be ballooned out to form a cardiac aneurysm and this is often lined with laminated thrombus. There may be fibrosis of the papillary muscles and in life this may have caused mitral reflux so that there may be some enlargement of the left atrium, and also some hypertrophy of the left ventricle.

Haemodynamics

The left ventricular end-diastolic pressure is raised and consequently the left atrial, pulmonary venous and pulmonary capillary pressures are raised also. The pulmonary artery pressure rises proportionately. Eventually the elevation of right sided pressures may be considerable and there may be salt and water retention with a picture of congestive failure.

Clinical features

There is usually a history of angina or one or more attacks of cardiac infarction. Following these there is often a history of progressive limitation of physical capacity owing to breathlessness or angina or both. There may be attacks of paroxysmal nocturnal dyspnoea and eventually oedema with the picture of congestive failure may develop. Sometimes fatigue with a sense of weakness or weariness of the limbs is a prominent symptom.

On examination in the earlier stages there may be a rather small volume pulse and the only other abnormal sign may be an atrial heart sound. If there is fibrosis of the papillary muscles mitral reflux may be present, shown by a systolic murmur which commonly begins in late systole and lasts until the second sound. In some cases, however, it may be mid-systolic or even pan-systolic (see p. 223). A cardiac aneurysm is indicated by the presence of a sustained cardiac impulse usually felt over rather a large area near or above the apex beat. There may be râles at the lung bases and in the later stages there may be congestive failure with a raised venous pressure, enlargement of the liver and dependent oedema.

The electrocardiogram

This may show signs of previous infarctions with abnormal Q waves and T wave inversions. Sometimes there is low voltage in which the sum of the QRS deflections in the limb leads is less than 15 mm. (p. 93).

Radiology

There may be enlargement of the heart with sometimes a discrete bulge due to a cardiac aneurysm. There is pulmonary venous engorgement and in the later stages there may be bilateral pleural effusions. In contrast to rheumatic heart disease, the size of the left atrium is no guide to the severity of mitral reflux due to ischaemia of the papillary muscles, presumably because the condition is of relatively short duration. The left atrium is at most only slightly enlarged. There is no calcium in the mitral valve and mitral reflux is best assessed by angiography. Coronary arteriography usually reveals serious disease in all three main branches.

Treatment

Coronary by-pass surgery may be considered for intractable angina. The risks are high if there is a raised left ventricular end-diastolic pressure and if the ventricular function on cine-angiography is seen to be poor with a small ejection fraction. Resection of a ventricular aneurysm occasionally may be combined with mitral valve replacement for mitral reflux due to papillary muscle fibrosis and is sometimes spectacularly successful in improving effort tolerance and even congestive heart failure. The aneurysm acts as a reservoir accepting a proportion of the left ventricular output and thus reduces the effective cardiac output. Its resection removes this handicap to the circulation and may possibly also increase the efficiency of left ventricular contraction.

Medical treatment is with nitrates, and beta-blockade provided heart failure is not severe. If heart failure threatens or is present then full digitalization is indicated (p. 295) together with diuretics.

FURTHER READING

Oliver, M., (1976) Dietary cholesterol, plasma cholesterol and coronary heart disease. *British Heart Journal*, **38**, 213.

Reports of Working Parties of Royal College of Physicians of London and British Cardiac Society:
  1. The life of the patient with coronary heart disease. (1975) *Journal of the Royal College of Physicians,* **10**, 5.
  2. Cardiac rehabilitation. (1975) *Journal of the Royal College of Physicians*, **9**, 281.
  3. Prevention of coronary disease (1976) *Journal of the Royal College of Physicians*, **10**, 213.

Sheldon, W.C., Rincon, G., Pichard, A., Razavi, M., Cheanvechai, C., & Loop, F.D. (1975) Surgical treatment of coronary artery disease. *Progress in Cardiovascular Disease,* **18**, 237.

Wood, P., (1969) *Disease of the Heart and Circulation*. London: Eyre and Spottiswoode.

12. Congenital Heart Disease

Introduction

Congenital heart disease may be due to abnormalities of development, maternal diseases during pregnancy (especially rubella), or intra-uterine disease of the fetus, but the first variety accounts for the majority of cases. Whatever the cause, the resulting malformations can be divided into two groups depending upon whether or not there is a defect allowing communication between the pulmonary and systemic circuits. Such a defect allows the current of blood to take a shortened pathway and this is called a *Shunt* as in electricity. If venous blood is shunted from the right heart or pulmonary artery into the systemic circuit, the arterial oxygen is reduced, *central cyanosis* results, and the pulmonary blood flow is *diminished*; by contrast, if arterial blood is shunted from the left heart or aorta into the pulmonary circuit, the arterial oxygen remains normal, there is *no cyanosis* and the pulmonary blood flow is *increased* at the expense of the systemic flow. The size and direction of flow through a Shunt depends on :–

1. The size of the defect.
2. The pressure difference across it.

This may be the normal pressure difference between the pulmonary and systemic circuits, or an abnormal one due to associated factors. Figure 12.1 shows four possibilities.

In (a) there is a left-to-right shunt across an atrial septal defect due to the normal pressure difference between the atria.

In (b) there is a left-to-right shunt across a ventricular septal defect; the right ventricular pressure is slightly raised due to the increased flow but the left ventricular pressure is much higher depending on the systemic blood pressure. Alterations in the latter will change the size of the shunt.

In (c) the intra-cardiac anatomy is the same but the shunt is in the reverse direction because the right ventricular pressure is raised as a result of narrowing of the pulmonary arterioles; the size of the shunt depends on the pulmonary vascular resistance which determines the right ventricular pressure.

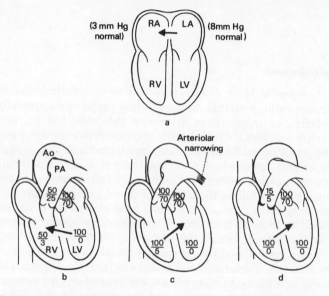

Fig. 12.1 Diagram illustrating the factors involved in intra-cardiac shunts. (a) Atrial septal defect. The left atrial pressure is normally higher than the right so that the shunt is from left to right. (b) Ventricular septal defect with left-to-right shunt and hyperkinetic pulmonary hypertension due to the increased flow. (c) Ventricular septal defect with right-to-left shunt due to high pulmonary vascular resistance (Eisenmenger Complex). (d) Ventricular septal defect with right-to-left shunt due to pulmonary stenosis (Tetralogy of Fallot). Some blood takes the path of least resistance through the defect and the ventricular pressures equalize.

In (d) the Shunt is also from right to left because the right ventricular pressure is raised as a result of pulmonary stenosis; the size of the Shunt depends on the severity of the obstruction.

It will now be apparent that although a defect between the pulmonary and systemic circuits is an unchanging anatomical fact, the pressure difference is a variable haemodynamic one and the Shunt can therefore change both in magnitude and direction with alteration of pressure relationships. The classification of congenital heart disease on the basis of the presence and direction of Shunts is therefore somewhat arbitrary, but these facts are of such crucial clinical importance that they must form the basis of any practical approach.

Treatment

Specific surgical treatment is now possible for certain types of congenital heart disease and this is described in the appropriate sections. Certain general measures are, however, applicable to all varieties. The patients are particularly prone to respiratory infections which may be unusually severe. Special precautions should be taken to avoid them and if they occur vigorous treatment with antibiotics should be given. Many varieties of congenital heart disease are susceptible to bacterial endocarditis and penicillin should be given for 5 days beginning on the day of any dental extraction. If effort dyspnoea is severe or if there is a risk of effort syncope, school games may have to be prohibited but attendance at a special school for physically handicapped children is rarely necessary.

Congenital heart disease with left ventricular hypertrophy and no shunt

Coarctation of the aorta (*Coarctus* means pressed together)

Morbid Anatomy. The abnormality consists of narrowing just distal to the left subclavian artery. There is commonly post-stenotic dilatation of the aorta beyond the coarctation and sometimes, dilatation proximal to it involving the origin of the left subclavian artery. The grade of narrowing ranges from barely perceptible to a pinhole orifice.

Haemodynamics. Alteration in the haemodynamics depends upon the grade of obstruction at the coarctation. If this is slight there may be no alteration: if however it is moderate or gross, there is a considerable systolic pressure gradient across the obstruction. There is hypertension in the upper part of the body and a reduced systolic pressure in the lower part. The hypertension is never extreme and never becomes 'malignant'. A collateral circulation develops by enlargement of vessels derived from the subclavian arteries, especially the internal mammaries, which link with the intercostals to maintain the blood flow to the lower half of the body. As a result of this, the mean aortic pressure distal to the obstruction may be scarcely reduced but pulsations in the main vessels of the legs are either delayed and weak, or impalpable.

Associated defects. The following may occur but only the first two are common:

1. Patent ductus arteriosus
2. Aortic stenosis or reflux
3. Bicuspid aortic valve
4. Mitral stenosis
5. Fibroelastosis

Clinical features. Severe coarctation may lead to left ventricular failure in infancy and this may be fatal. Otherwise symptoms are slight although adults may complain of undue fatigue in the legs. On examination a well-developed upper half of the body may be found, contrasting with slender legs. There is exaggerated arterial pulsation in the suprasternal notch and this sign in children or young adults is practically pathognomonic of coarctation and should lead immediately to palpation of the femoral arteries in which pulsation will be found to be weak and delayed or absent. Collateral vessels are most easily found if the patient is asked to face the examiner and touch his toes. If the patient is placed between a good light and the clinician, the vessels are thrown into relief and cast easily visible shadows. There is moderate hypertension in the arms and a lower pressure in the legs (the reverse of normal). There is also some left ventricular hypertrophy and a systolic murmur over the mid-chest. If the left ventricular hypertrophy is moderate or considerable and there is a loud mid-systolic murmur at the base of the heart radiating to the neck, associated aortic stenosis should be suspected. In the interscapular area the systolic murmur is late and may be due to flow through the coarctation. A systolic or continuous murmur may be heard over collateral vessels, and a continuous murmur at the second left space suggests a patent ductus.

The cardiogram. This may show increased voltage in the limb leads, a deep S in V1 and tall R in V6. S–T–T depression suggests an associated aortic valve abnormality.

Complications. Bacterial infection is a rare complication but cerebral or sub-arachnoid haemorrhage may occur from an associated congenital weakness of cerebral arteries.

Treatment. If heart failure occurs in infancy surgical resection should be performed immediately after an intensive course of medical treatment. Otherwise patients with well developed signs of the abnormality should be operated on in their teens or early adult life. Those with normal blood pressure, and palpable although delayed femoral pulses, may require no treatment.

Congenital aortic stenosis

Morbid anatomy. In some cases the valve cusps are fused together forming a membrane with a central orifice, perhaps as result of fetal endocarditis; in others the valve is bicuspid due to a developmental abnormality, and gradually becomes thickened, calcified and narrowed. The disorder is sometimes familial.

Haemodynamics. There is a pressure gradient across the valve ranging between 30 to 150 mmHg or more.

Clinical features. Most patients have no symptoms but severe cases have angina or effort syncope. The physical signs include a small volume pulse which is sometimes slow-rising, and left ventricular hypertrophy. There is a rasping mid-systolic murmur often with a thrill at the second right space and in the neck. The murmur may also be heard at the left sternal edge and the cardiac apex. Splitting of the second sound may be reversed—the obstruction to the left ventricular outflow delaying the aortic valve closure until after pulmonary closure has occurred.

The cardiogram. In severe cases leads V4 to 6 show increased voltage and eventually T wave inversion.

Radiology. The heart size may be normal, since the hypertrophy is concentric, but post-stenotic dilatation of the aorta may be seen (Fig. 4.5a).

Prognosis. There is a risk of sudden death on exertion at any time and perhaps it is greatest in unsuspected cases in childhood when sudden violent physical exertion is frequently undertaken. Attempts have been made to estimate this risk and the results in children range from 1 to 7 per cent the average being about 2 to 3 per cent.

Treatment. As operative treatment requires cardio-pulmonary by-pass and carries a mortality of at least 5 per cent it clearly cannot be advised for all children. Moreover, valvotomy is usually followed by some reflux and invariably by restenosis with calcification later, so that ultimately valve-replacement becomes necessary. Therefore, it seems reasonable, to defer operation as long as possible and to apply the criteria used in adults, namely angina, dyspnoea, effort syncope and increasing left ventricular dominance in the cardiogram, and a pressure gradient exceeding 80 mm Hg for advising operative treatment. Meanwhile competitive games and sudden violent exertion must be prohibited.

Fibroelastosis

Definition. A form of congenital or neonatal heart disease of unknown aetiology characterized by thickening of the endocardium of the ventricles with fibrous and elastic tissue which may involve the mitral and tricuspid or other valves.

The condition may be subdivided into two groups, according to the presence or absence of associated congenital abnormalities of the heart. If present, these dominate the clinical picture which is described under the heading of the defect concerned. This section deals only with the isolated abnormality.

Clinical features. Heart failure with or without signs of mitral or tricuspid reflux occurs in the first few months of life, with failure to thrive, feeding difficulites, tachypnoea, liver enlargement and tachycardia. The illness may be fulminating, when death occurs within a few days, or it may last weeks or months.

Treatment. There may be a dramatic response to full digitalization and diuretics and this has reduced the mortality from over 80 per cent to about 20 per cent. The survivors may well have normal life expectancy and they certainly appear to be normal in childhood.

Congenital heart disease with right ventricular hypertrophy and no shunt

Congenital Pulmonary Stenosis

Morbid anatomy. There are two pathological types—valvar and infundibular. The valvar type may result from a developmental abnormality of the cusps or perhaps from an intrauterine inflammation. In place of the normal cusps there is a dome-shaped membrane with a small central hole measuring 1 to 5 mm. The infundibular type is much less common, and the obstruction is produced by a muscular or membranous ridge situated below a normal pulmonary valve.

Haemodynamics. The gradient across the pulmonary valve ranges from 30 to 100 mmHg or more and on catheterization the transition from low to high pressure is found to occur abruptly at the valve in pulmonary valve stenosis but lower and more gradually in the body of the right ventricle in infundibular stenosis (Fig. 12.2). In very severe cases the right ventricular diastolic pressure is also raised and consequently the right atrial pressure rises too. This may open the foramen ovale with the production of a right-to-left interatrial shunt and cyanosis.

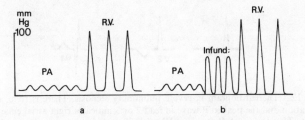

Fig. 12.2 Pressures recorded during withdrawal of the catheter from pulmonary artery to right ventricle. (a) Pulmonary valve stenosis. The pressure changes abruptly from a low pressure in the pulmonary artery to a high pressure in the right ventricle. (b) Infundibular and pulmonary valve stenosis. There is a zone of intermediate systolic pressure between the low pressure in the pulmonary artery and the high pressure in the ventricle.

Clinical features. Mild or moderate cases have no symptoms but in severe cases there may be effort dyspnoea, syncope or angina (see p. 150). Usually there is no cyanosis and the patient is well grown. The peripheral pulses are small in volume but the 'a' waves of the jugular pulse are exaggerated and characteristic "giant 'a' waves" may be seen. There is right ventricular hypertrophy and a loud rasping mid-systolic murmur usually with a thrill at the second left interspace close to the sternum. The murmur may be preceded by an ejection click and followed by a widely split second sound, the pulmonary component of which is extremely quiet.

The cardiogram. This is normal in mild cases but with increasing severity there may be tall pointed P waves due to atrial hypertrophy, increasing right axis deviation and exaggeration of the R wave in V1 with ST–T depression in leads V1 to V4 (Fig. 12.3).

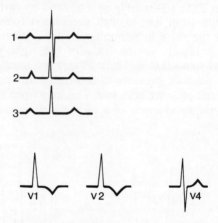

Fig. 12.3 The cardiogram in severe pulmonary stenosis. There is right axis deviation and the peaked P wave in lead 2 or 3 indicates right atrial enlargement. The dominant R wave in V1 with T wave inversion is due to right ventricular hypertrophy.

Radiology. There is post-stenotic dilatation of the main and left pulmonary arteries (except in cases of infundibular stenosis) due to turbulence produced by the jet of blood from the narrowed pulmonary valve orifice (Fig. 12.4).

Treatment. Patients with syncope, angina, or marked right ventricular dominance in the cardiogram, or a gradient of over 60 mmHg should have surgical treatment. The valve is exposed by opening the pulmonary artery under cardio-pulmonary by-pass and the membranous valve is incised along the presumed lines of the commisures. The mortality is low (about 1 to 2 per cent) and the results good. Infundibular stenosis requires resection of the fibrous or muscular narrowing.

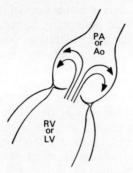

Fig. 12.4 The mechanism of post-stenotic dilatation. The narrow jet from the stenotic valve produces excessive turbulence just above the valve and dilatation of the vessel occurs in this position.

Congenital heart disease with left-to-right shunt and left ventricular hypertrophy

Patent ductus arteriosus

Morbid anatomy. The ductus arteriosus connects the isthmus of the aorta to the left pulmonary artery and normally closes at or shortly after birth by a process of endarteritis. Maternal rubella in the first trimester commonly results in persistent patency often associated with cataract and deafness. Administration of a high concentration of oxygen in the neonatal period may delay closure. A patent ductus may be associated with other abnormalities but here only the isolated anomaly will be considered.

Haemodynamics. Oxygenated blood passes from the high pressure systemic circuit through the ductus into the low pressure pulmonary circuit in the majority of cases, and cardiac catheterization shows oxygen saturation at least 10 per cent higher in pulmonary artery blood than in the right ventricle. The pulmonary blood flow may be three to four times the systemic flow, and this large volume passes to the lungs and returns to the left side of the heart for the circuit to be completed. The left atrium and left ventricle are therefore dilated and hypertrophied. The pulmonary artery pressure is raised only proportionately to the increased flow and the pulmonary resistance remains normal owing to arteriolar dilatation (hyperkinetic pulmonary hypertension). In about 15 per cent of cases this dilatation does not occur and obstructive pulmonary hypertension results with possible reversal of the shunt (see Eisenmenger syndrome, p. 193).

Clinical features. Females are affected twice as commonly as males. In infancy the abrupt physiological reduction in pulmonary vascular resistance at, or shortly after birth, allows the sudden development of a large left-right shunt which may precipitate left ventricular failure. If this is survived or does not occur, symptoms of dyspnoea are relatively slight in childhood but become more conspicuous in later life.

On examination the signs common to all varieties of 'aortic leak' are found, including warm hands, 'water-hammer' pulses, capillary pulsation and a hyperkinetic left ventricle. The characteristic sign, without which the diagnosis cannot be made without special investigations, *is a continuous murmur*. This has a rumbling, roaring or 'machinery' quality and is best heard in the second left space where there is often a thrill. A loud split second sound with a peculiar clattering quality can also be heard during the loudest portion of the murmur. The increased blood flow through the left heart commonly gives rise to a delayed diastolic 'flow murmur' from the mitral valve, especially in children. The characteristic continuous murmur is quite often absent in infancy, when there may be merely a mid-systolic murmur at the base. It may also be absent if the shunt is limited by pulmonary hypertension. In such cases cardiac catheterization is required to establish the diagnosis.

The cardiogram. This may be normal or show increased voltage in limb and chest leads but the T waves are upright.

Radiology. The left ventricle is hypertrophied and enlarged; the aorta and pulmonary arteries are prominent and unduly pulsatile, and there is pulmonary plethora.

Treatment. If there is heart failure in infancy intensive medical treatment is required and surgical closure should be carried out as soon as improvement is judged to be maximal.

Otherwise ligation should be deferred until the child is two years old and may be undertaken at any time after this into late adult life. As the operation carries a low risk (1 to 2 per cent) and abolishes both left ventricular hypertrophy and the risk of bacterial infection, it should always be advised unless there is serious pulmonary hypertension. If the pulmonary vascular resistance is high but the shunt is predominantly left-to-right surgical treatment may be advised although the risks are high. However, if the shunt is predominantly right-to-left with cyanosis, surgical treatment is contra-indicated.

Congenital heart disease with left-to-right shunt and right ventricular hypertrophy

Atrial septal defect

Morbid anatomy. The commonest type of atrial septal defect is a deficiency in the septum secondum in the region of the fossa ovalis (it is not merely patency of the foramen ovale). The defect usually measures 2 to 4 cm in diameter, and it may be associated with anomalous pulmonary veins draining into the right atrium.

Much less common is a defect in the septum primum resulting in an orifice situated just above the atrio-ventricular ring and often associated with defects of the mitral or tricuspid valves which may be incompetent(Fig. 12.5).

Haemodynamics. The mean left atrial pressure is normally 5 mmHg greater than the right atrial pressure and consequently an atrial septal defect allows a left-to-right interatrial shunt. It follows that the amount of blood passing to the lungs is greater than that passing to the systemic circulation and the ratio of the pulmonary to systemic flow is commonly 2:1 or more. As a result the right atrium, right ventricle and pulmonary arteries are considerably dilated and hypertrophied. Usually the pulmonary vessels dilate to accept this increased flow and the pulmonary vascular resistance is normal. In only about six per cent of cases is it raised, when reversal of the shunt may occur.

Clinical features of the ostium secundum type. Females are affected three times as often as males. Symptoms do not usually occur until the fourth or fifth decade and consist of

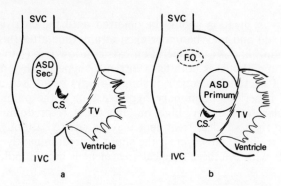

Fig. 12.5 Diagram of the ostium primum and ostium secondum types of atrial septal defect (ASD). The commoner secundum type in which the defect is in the position of the fossa ovalis is shown in (a). In the less common primum type shown in (b) the defect is close to the atrio-ventricular valves which may be deformed. SVC = Superior vena cava; RA = Right atrium; CS = Coronary sinus; TV = Tricuspid valve.

effort dyspnoea possibly with palpitations due to atrial fibrillation. This is the only form of congenital heart disease in which this dysrhythmia commonly occurs.

On examination the jugular venous pressure and pulse are usually normal unless there is fibrillation, when CV waves may be seen. The peripheral pulse is small in volume and palpation of the chest discloses a hyperkinetic right ventricle, often with a palpable thrust over the pulmonary artery. There is a mid-systolic murmur in the parasternal region but there is no clearly localized point of maximal intensity and no thrill. There is also wide and constant splitting of the second sound and the increased flow through the right heart may result in a functional diastolic murmur from the tricuspid valve audible between the xiphisternum and the apex.

Cardiogram. There is usually right axis deviation and lead V1 almost invariably shows an RSR' complex (Fig. 12.6). The diagnosis is almost untenable in the absence of the latter.

Radiology. There is enlargement of the right atrium, the right ventricle and the pulmonary artery and its branches which can be seen on radioscopy to pulsate vigorously.

Treatment. Operative closure should be advised in almost

all cases as the risks are very low and the results excellent. After operation many patients who were previously 'asymptomatic' discover unfamiliar vigour and capacity for effort.

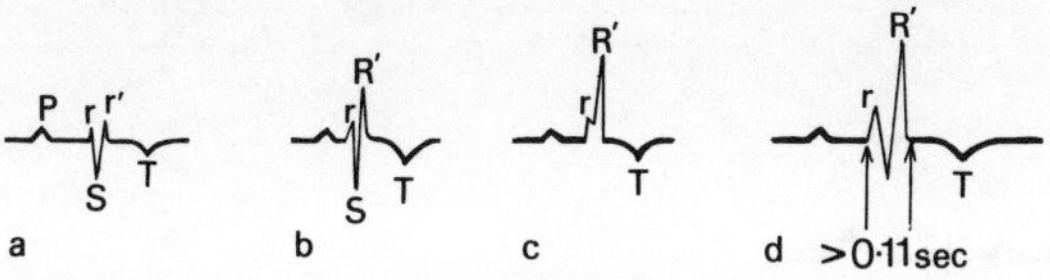

Fig. 12.6 The cardiogram in atrial septal defect showing varieties of the rSr' complex in V1. In (a), (b) and (c) the duration of the QRS complex is within normal limits and the height of the secondary 'R' wave is related to the degree of right ventricular hypertrophy. In (d) the QRS duration exceeds 0.11 sec indicating right bundle branch block. The height of the 'R' wave is then unrelated to the degree of hypertrophy.

Clinical features of ostium primum type. This variety differs in the following respects from the commoner ostium secundum type. First, symptoms occur earlier and there is a greater risk of pulmonary hypertension. Secondly, in addition to the mid-systolic murmur, there may be pan-systolic murmurs due to mitral or tricuspid reflux. Thirdly, the cardiogram characteristically shows *left axis deviation with a deep broad S wave in leads 2 and 3 together with RSR' complexes in lead 1* (Fig. 12.7). Finally operative treatment is more difficult and carries a higher risk but is nevertheless advisable as the prognosis is worse than in the secundum type of defect.

Congenital heart disease with left to right shunt and combined ventricular hypertrophy

Ventricular septal defect

Morbid anatomy. The defect usually occurs in the membranous portion of the inter-ventricular septum or in the muscular portion just below this. Its diameter varies from a few millimetres to several centimetres but is usually between 1–3 centimetres.

Haemodynamics. As the left ventricular pressure normally exceeds the right, there is a left-to-right inter-ventricular shunt and the pulmonary blood flow is consequently increased. The pulmonary to systemic flow ratio is commonly 2–4/1. It will

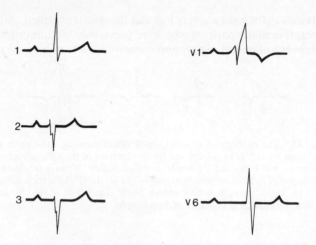

Fig. 12.7 The cardiogram in ostium primum atrial septal defect. There is left axis deviation with a deep notched S wave in lead 2. Right ventricular hypertrophy is indicated by the rsR' complex, tall R' wave, and inverted T wave in V1.

be appreciated that both ventricles are performing increased work as a result of the exaggerated pulmonary blood flow and both are therefore dilated and hypertrophied. The pulmonary vascular resistance is increased in only about 15 per cent of cases. In these the right ventricular pressure may equal the left and a bidirectional shunt occurs (see the Eisenmenger Complex, p. 193).

Clinical features. These depend on the size of the orifice and the pulmonary vascular resistance. A tiny defect produces no symptoms—The *'Maladie de Roger',* whereas a larger defect of a centimetre or more may cause heart failure in infancy, as the physiological fall of the pulmonary vascular resistance after birth abruptly allows a large left-to-right shunt with overloading of the right ventricle. The infant ceases to feed properly, develops tachypnoea, tachycardia and liver enlargement. However, this occurs in only a proportion of cases and in the remainder, symptoms are delayed until childhood or adult life when effort dyspnoea may be noticed.

On examination the venous pressure is normal but the arterial pulse is small. The heart is hyperkinetic to palpation and pulsation of the pulmonary artery may be felt in the second left space. There is a pan-systolic murmur and usually a thrill in the parasternal region, and the second sound is split. The murmur has a well-localized point of maximal intensity in the third and fourth interspaces as described by Roger, and this is the only physical sign in cases with a small defect.

The cardiogram. This commonly shows an RSR' complex in lead V1 due to the dilated right ventricle and a tall R wave with upright T in lead V5 due to the enlarged left ventricle.

Radioscopy. There is enlargement of both ventricles and of the main pulmonary arteries, which pulsate with abnormal amplitude. There is pulmonary plethora, but the aorta is small. In cases with a very small defect the cardiac outlines are normal and the pulmonary vasculature is normal.

Prognosis. The Maladie de Roger has a nearly normal life expectancy although there is a very small risk of bacterial endocarditis. With large defects the mortality is high in infancy and may reach fifty per cent if there is heart failure. However, if the first twelve months are survived, many patients reach adult life or even middle age, though it remains uncertain why so few adults are seen with moderate sized defects.

Treatment. Treatment is determined by the size of the shunt, the pulmonary vascular resistance, and the balance between the shortened expectation of life and the risks of operation. The *Maladie de Roger* requires no treatment and no restrictions. At the other extreme are patients with considerable or gross enlargement of the heart, pulmonary flow more than twice the systemic flow and near equalisation of the right and left ventricular pressures due to the large pulmonary flow and not to increased pulmonary vascular resistance. These patients certainly have a diminished expectation of life and operation should be advised. Between these two extremes there are patients with few or no symptoms, only slight to moderate enlargement of the heart, a considerable shunt but a right ventricular pressure of not more than about half the systemic pressure and low pulmonary vascular resistance. Because operation carries an appreciable morbidity, with risk of heart block through damage to the bundle of His, incomplete closure of the defect and possible subsequent infection, and also because it is not known whether closure improves life expectancy, operation is not usually advised in these cases at the present time.

In infancy heart failure may occur when the pulmonary resistance abruptly drops during the first few weeks and months of life with the development of a huge left to right shunt. These patients need urgent treatment with digoxin and diuretics.

If the response is not thoroughly satisfactory, the operation of 'banding' the pulmonary artery may be advised. The pulmonary artery is narrowed by tying a ligature round it to produce a partial obstruction and elevation of the right ventricular pressure. This diminishes the left-to-right shunt and may tide the infant over a critical period until operative closure of the defect can be performed with an acceptable risk.

The differential diagnosis of parasternal systolic murmurs without cyanosis

The diagnosis usually rests between the following conditions:
1. Physiological systolic murmurs of childhood.
2. Atrial septal defect.
3. Pulmonary stenosis.
4. Ventricular septal defect.
5. Aortic stenosis.

1. *Physiological murmurs of childhood.*

There are no relevant symptoms or cardiac signs apart from a murmur occupying early and mid-systole heard in the parasternal region. There is no definite point of maximum intensity and splitting of the second heart sound is normal. The phonocardiogram shows a shortened interval between the first heart sound and beginning of the carotid pulse upstroke indicating unusually rapid development of maximum intraventricular pressure. The rapid acceleration of the ejected blood produces a murmur early in the ejection phase. The shortened pre-ejection period returns to normal at puberty when the murmur disappears.

2. *Atrial septal defect*

The characteristics of the murmur are somewhat similar to

those of the physiological murmur of childhood as it is due to increased volume and velocity of flow in the pulmonary artery but the heart is hyperkinetic to palpation and the second sound is widely and constantly split. The cardiogram and X-ray are confirmatory.

3. *Pulmonary stenosis*

There is right ventricular hypertrophy but the heart is hyperdynamic—the pulsation is forceful but small in amplitude. The murmur is usually mid-systolic but may reach the aortic component of the second sound and the maximum intensity is well localized at the second left space with a thrill. The second sound may be single, or split with an extremely quiet delayed pulmonary component. The cardiogram shows right ventricular hypertrophy.

4. *Ventricular septal defect*

Although the murmur may be widespread there is usually a small area in the third or fourth left interspaces where it is undoubtedly louder than anywhere else, and the thrill is also maximum there. The second sound is less widely split than in atrial sept defect and the heart is hyperkinetic (large amplitude pulsation). The cardiogram shows combined right and left ventricular hypertrophy.

5. *Aortic stenosis*

There is a normal or exaggerated left ventricular impulse and the rasping mid-systolic murmur may be loudest in the parasternal region rather than the 2nd right space. It may also be heard in the neck. A thrill may be felt in either or both positions.

The salient features in differentiation are summarized in Table 12.1.

Congenital heart disease with right-to-left shunt, low pulmonary blood flow and high pulmonary vascular resistance

Eisenmenger's Complex and The Eisenmenger syndrome

Introduction. Eisenmenger described a *complex* with ventricular septal defect enlarged pulmonary artery (due to pulmonary hypertension), right ventricular hypertrophy, and 'over-riding' aorta. The high pulmonary vascular resistance causes a right-to-left shunt across the ventricular septal defect

Table 12.1

Parasternal systolic murmurs

Characteristics	Childhood murmur	A.S.D.	P.S.	V.S.D.	Aortic stenosis
		No cyanosis			
Timing	Early–mid-systolic	mid-systolic	mid-systolic	pan-systolic	mid-systolic
Area of max: intensity	Large	Large	small	small	small
Site	parasternal	parasternal	2nd left space	3–4 left space	Parasternal & often 2nd right space
Thrill	no	no	usual	usual	usual
2nd sound	normal split	constant split	split; quiet pulm;	split	may be normal
Palpation	normal	hyperkinetic R.V.	hyperdynamic R.V.	hyperkinetic R.V. & L.V.	normal or L.V. +
E.C.G.	normal	V.1 rSr' or rSR'	V.1 R > S or Normal	VI rSr' V5 Tall R or normal	normal or L.A.D. or L.V.H.
X-ray; Lungs.	normal	plethora	oligaemic	plethora	normal

with consequent cyanosis (Fig. 12.1c). However a closely similar picture of cyanosis with signs of pulmonary hypertension can be produced by other malformations and it is therefore convenient to consider them as a group under the general heading of The Eisenmenger *syndrome* which may be defined as follows:

A clinical syndrome of Cyanotic Congenital Heart Disease due to a right-to-left or bidirectional shunt produced by a raised pulmonary vascular resistance at or above systemic level.

The commonest malformations producing this syndrome are ventricular septal defect (the original *Eisenmenger complex*), patent ductus arteriosus and atrial septal defect. Less common causes include transposition of the great vessels, single ventricle, truncus arteriosus, single atrium and total anomalous pulmonary venous drainage.

Haemodynamics. At birth there is normally a precipitous fall of pulmonary vascular resistance as the lungs are aerated and the pulmonary blood vessels unfurl. This allows a large left-to-right shunt through any of the defects mentioned above and hyperkinetic pulmonary hypertension occurs at once. Sometimes this seems to prevent any further relaxation of arteriolar tone and the pulmonary vascular resistance fails to fall to normal levels. Intimal thickening of the arterioles follows quickly and the pulmonary vascular resistance may rise still higher causing reversal of the shunt.

It is not known why this sequence of changes occurs in only a proportion of cases—about fifteen per cent of cases of ventricular septal defect and patent ductus. However, the lower incidence of six per cent in atrial septal defect *is* explicable. The normal thick wall of the right ventricle in infancy is uncompliant and resists filling from the right atrium. This limits the left-to-right inter-atrial shunt in early life and usually allows the normal relaxation of arteriolar tone to occur. In all types of Eisenmenger syndrome the rise of pulmonary vascular resistance to systemic level usually occurs in early infancy or childhood and is irreversible. It is rare to *observe* a change from hyperkinetic pulmonary hypertension to the Eisenmenger syndrome.

Clinical features. There is cyanosis and effort dyspnoea but squatting is uncommon. Examination reveals right ventricular hypertrophy and the second sound is usually split. If the syndrome is caused by a patent ductus arteriosus the legs may be bluer than the arms owing to the site of the shunt and there may be a water-hammer pulse suggesting that the shunt is bi-directional. If a ventricular septal defect is the cause squatting is sometimes seen. In cases due to atrial septal defect giant A waves may be present and right ventricular hypertrophy is extreme.

The cardiogram. This shows right ventricular hypertrophy but some left-sided enlargement is suggested by the presence of Q waves in V5 in cases due to patent ductus and ventricular septal defect.

Radiology. If the syndrome is caused by a patent ductus or ventricular septal defect the heart is moderately enlarged but if atrial septal defect is the cause the heart is huge. A right aortic arch suggests a ventricular septal defect, while a huge pulmonary artery suggests a patent ductus or atrial septal defect as the cause of the syndrome.

Differential diagnosis. Differentiation from conditions with *low and normal pulmonary artery pressure group* depends upon recognition of pulmonary hypertension by the loud pulmonary component of a split second sound and perhaps palpable pulsation of the pulmonary artery. Radiologically the enlarged *main* branches contrasting with scanty peripheral markings suggests the diagnosis. Recognition of the type of malformation causing the syndrome involves consideration of the rarities mentioned on page 195 and demands exact determination of the site or sites of the shunt and delineation of the anatomy by catheterization and angiocardiography.

Right-to-left shunt with right ventricular hypertrophy and low pulmonary flow and pressure

Tetralogy of Fallot

Morbid anatomy. This complex consists of a ventricular septal defect, dextroposition of the aorta, pulmonary stenosis and consequent right ventricular hypertrophy. There is usually thickening of the infundibular muscle and this forms the main obstruction to right ventricular outflow, and sometimes produces a distinct infundibular chamber. Pulmonary valve stenosis forms a second but usually lesser obstruction (Fig.

12.8). Sometimes, however, the whole of the right ventricular outflow tract including the pulmonary valve ring is hypoplastic.

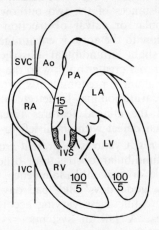

Fig. 12.8 A diagram of the Tetralogy of Fallot. There is pulmonary valve stenosis an infundibular chamber (I) and infundibular stenosis (IVS). The obstructions cause some blood to take the path of lower resistance through the ventricular septal defect to the aorta, and the interventricular pressures are equal.

Haemodynamics. As usual, these depend chiefly upon resistance relationships and the degree of dextroposition of the aorta is of secondary importance. It will be seen from the diagram that the right ventricle has alternative exit pathways, namely the pulmonary artery and the ventricular septal defect. If the pulmonary infundibular obstruction is severe the right ventricular pressure equals the left and blood passes more easily to the aorta than to the pulmonary artery producing considerable cyanosis and a low pulmonary flow; a drop in systemic resistance will further increase the right-to-left shunt. However, if the pulmonary obstruction is slighter, more blood will pass into the pulmonary artery than into the aorta, and cyanosis will be less severe. If the obstruction is mainly due to muscular hypertrophy of the infundibulum, it may vary from hour to hour or day to day with consequent variation in cyanosis. This type can be influenced by beta-blockade. The left ventricle also has alternative outlets through the septal defect or into the aorta. The route taken, again depends on the relative resistances of the two outflow pathways. With severe infundibular or valvar obstruction or low systemic resistance, outflow to the aorta is encouraged. By contrast, if there is only slight infundibular obstruction and higher systemic resistance a greater outflow to the pulmonary artery ensues, and the shunt is predominantly left-to-right. In these cases arterial desaturation may be detected only by laboratory estimation and the clinical features resemble those of a ventricular septal defect with small left-to-right shunt.

Clinical features. Cyanosis is present from birth in cases with severe infundibular obstruction, otherwise it may be delayed for weeks or even until adolescence. Characteristically the patient has 'good days' and 'bad days'—the degree of cyanosis and breathlessness varying according to the outflow resistances. A fall in systemic resistance allows a greater right-to-left shunt and consequently a smaller pulmonary flow with anoxia and dyspnoea. This may cause powerful contraction of the infundibulum which makes the obstruction worse and a severe cyanotic attack results. Squatting on effort is particularly common in this malformation. This posture increases the venous return to the right ventricle which contracts more powerfully according to Starling's law and increases pulmonary flow. It also raises the systemic pressure limiting the right-to-left shunt and facilitates respiratory excursions.

On examination cyanosis is commonly obvious in the tongue and there is finger clubbing. The jugular venous pressure is normal but there is a gentle parasternal thrust due to right ventricular hypertrophy. There is usually a parasternal systolic murmur with a thrill, although this may be absent in infancy, and the second sound is usually single owing to the low pulmonary artery pressure. Severe cases with intense cyanosis may have continuous murmurs over the front or back of the chest. These are due to blood flow through bronchial arteries which enlarge to carry blood to the oligaemic lungs. Heart failure does not occur probably because the right ventricle has an escape route into the aorta.

In some cases cyanosis is minimal and the clinical picture

resembles that of a ventricular septal defect.

The cardiogram. This shows right axis deviation and a dominant R in V1. Extreme right ventricular hypertrophy is unusual as the right ventricular pressure cannot rise above systemic level.

Radiology. The heart is characteristically normal in size but not in shape often having the typical appearances of a Dutch clog or Sabot (Fig. 12.9). The pulmonary vascular markings are sparse and a right aortic arch supports the diagnosis.

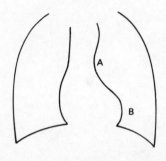

Fig. 12.9 The radiological appearances in the Tetralogy of Fallot. There is a deep pulmonary bay (A) and a tip-tilted apex producing the sabot appearance (B). The heart size is normal.

Differential diagnosis. The features described usually make the diagnosis relatively easy on clinical grounds alone.

Treatment. Cyanotic attacks in infancy may be due to contraction of the hypertrophied infundibulum which can often be relieved by beta-blockade with propranolol. The persistant source of disability, however, is the low pulmonary blood flow which can be improved by Blalock's operation in which the subclavian artery is anastomosed to the pulmonary artery. The risks are relatively slight and the results good for many years. In severe cases this operation can be used as a palliative measure until the child is fit to undergo closure of the septal defect and resection of the pulmonary stenosis— an operation which carries an appreciably higher mortality at the present time.

FURTHER READING

Keith, J.D., Rose, V., Collins, G., & Kidd, B.S.L. (1971) Ventricular septal defect. Incidence morbidity mortality in various age groups. *British Heart Journal,* **33** (suppl), 81.

McNamara, D.G. & Mullins, C.E. (1971) Diagnosis of congenital heart disease in acyanotic infants. *Progress in Cardiovascular Disease,* **14**, 81.

Griffiths, Sylvia P. & Ellis, K. (1974) Differential diagnosis of cyanotic congenital heart disease. *Progress in Cardiovascular Disease,* **14,** 93.

Nadas, A.S. & Fyler, D.C. (1972) *Paediatric Cardiology.* London: W.B. Saunders.

13. Rheumatic Fever

Definition

Rheumatic fever is a systemic disorder probably caused by an abnormal response to streptococcal infection. It is characterized by malaise sometimes with fever, and *one or more* of the following features: polyarthritis, carditis, subcutaneous nodules, chorea and erythema marginatum.

Aetiology

In many cases a throat infection with group A haemolytic streptococci precedes the onset of the disease by ten to twenty days. The serum anti-streptolysin titre (AST) and ESR are naturally raised during the infection but instead of returning to normal, they remain high until the onset of the disease. In other cases the raised AST at the onset of rheumatic fever points to a previous subclinical streptococcal infection.

There is a hereditary predisposition and often familial incidence of the disease which is especially common in poor and overcrowded communities. It usually occurs between the ages of three and twenty-five but may be seen up to the age of sixty or even later. In Europe and North America it has become progressively milder in severity and less common during the last 10 to 15 years.

Pathology

The characteristic lesion is the Aschoff node which occurs in connective tissue and consists of a central area of necrosis in the collagen surrounded by multinucleated giant cells, plasma cells, lymphocytes and fibroblasts. These lesions occur in connective tissue in close relation to small arterioles. They are common in the pericardium and other serous surfaces and a few may be seen in the connective tissue septa among the muscle bundles of the heart. In this situation however, they are scanty and damage to muscle fibres is conspicuous by its absence.

In the active phase of the disease the heart valves may become oedematous and the endocardium is damaged along the contact margins 2 or 3 millimetres from the free edges. At this site tiny vegetations are formed consisting of platelet thrombi. When the underlying inflammation subsides fibrosis and contraction follow while similar changes cause shortening of the chordae tendineae. The site of these lesions at the contact points of the cusps suggests that trauma determines the position of the damage. This is also indicated by the relative frequency with which the various valves are involved. The mitral valve closing at the highest pressure—about 100 mm Hg is subjected to the greatest stress and is the most frequently affected; the aortic valve closing at systemic diastolic pressure is the second most commonly involved; the tricuspid valve which closes at the right ventricular systolic pressure of about 20 mmHg is infrequently affected and the pulmonary valve which closes at about a pressure of 10 mm Hg is almost never affected. It follows that aortic valve disease is usually accompanied by mitral disease, and tricuspid involvement is usually accompanied by disease of both the aortic and mitral valves.

During the active phase of the disorder, distortion of the cusps and weakening of the mitral valve ring leads to mitral reflux causing left ventricular dilatation and this in turn interferes with the normal function of the papillary muscles causing still more reflux (p. 221). The jet of regurgitated blood from the left ventricle strikes the posterior wall of the left atrium and this trauma determines the development of a necrotic area in the atrium in which numerous Aschoff bodies may be found.

Involvement of the aortic valve also leads to reflux and dilatation of the left ventricle. It is probable that any change in the heart size observed in the acute phase of the disease is explicable by dilatation due to leaky valves, and evidence of *direct* involvement of the heart muscle with consequent impairment of its function is weak.

Pericardial involvement may result in a fibrous pericarditis with a loculated effusion which is usually small in quantity. It should be noted that although the mitral valve may become leaky early in the acute phase of the disease, stenosis, due to fibrosis and adhesion of the commissures, takes at least five years to develop.

Clinical features

The younger the patient the more severe is the disease. The onset in young children was often acute with fever, malaise, anorexia and sometimes epistaxis, but as the disease has become milder a gradual onset with lassitude and loss of weight has become commoner. Even when fever and arthritis are absent however, carditis can occur. Usually one or more of the following features are found:

Migratory arthritis

Characteristically pain occurs in one of the larger joints such as the elbow, wrist, shoulder, knee, ankle or hip and persists for two or three days before gradually diminishing, when another of these joints may be involved. Redness or swelling is unusual but the pain may be sufficiently severe to prevent the child from moving the limb or walking, but a 'pseudo-paralysis' or such severe pain in one hip as to lead to suspicion of suppurative arthritis or osteomyelitis, is now rare. The features of the arthritis are similar to those which may follow dysentery or gonococcal infection in which an allergic mechanism is also probable.

Carditis

This used to occur in about fifty per cent of children with rheumatic fever but is now less common and still more rare in adults. The more florid the general clinical manifestations of the disease the more likely it is to occur, but when chorea is the sole clinical feature, evidence of carditis is infrequent. The five most reliable signs of carditis are as follows:

1. *Mitral valvitis.* The most dependable sign of mitral valve involvement is a quiet, low-pitched delayed diastolic murmur following directly on the third heart sound. It is sharply localized and best heard with a bell chest piece with the patient in the left lateral position. The mode of production of the

murmur, which may persist for only a few days or weeks, is uncertain. Perhaps oedema limits the mobility of the cusps which fail to open fully in diastole and therefore vibrate in the blood stream during the rapid filling phase of the ventricle. In many cases the murmur does not entirely disappear; it can be made evident by exercise and over the years develops into the murmur of mitral stenosis.

If an apical pan-systolic murmur is observed to develop during the course of the illness it is also evidence of carditis. It is due to mitral reflux, either from involvement of the valve and valve ring, or a secondary effect of aortic reflux which causes left ventricular dilatation with consequent impairment of papillary muscle function. (p. 221).

Apical systolic murmurs must be differentiated from those which occur occasionally in other infections or in fevers without carditis. Such murmurs are usually neither loud nor rough in quality and in general the seriousness of the systolic murmur is proportional to its loudness.

2. *Aortic reflux*. This may occur in the first few weeks of rheumatic fever and results in the characteristic murmur best heard along the left sternal border.

3. *Cardiographic abnormalities*. Partial atrio-ventricular block is indicated by prolongation of the P–R interval in the cardiogram beyond the normal limits for the age of the patient; it occurs transiently in less than ten per cent of cases of rheumatic fever. Prolongation of the Q–T interval may also occur but is a less reliable sign of carditis. It must be corrected for the heart rate by dividing by the square root of the cycle length.

4. *Pericarditis*. Pericarditis is an indication of a severe attack and is now rare. It may occur at any time during the first few weeks of the illness and is usually marked by a sudden deterioration with higher fever, white cell count and ESR. There is pericardial friction and some effusion may develop but never enough to merit aspiration. It may neverthless produce a sudden increase in the size of the heart shadow on chest X-ray and may cause compression collapse of the lower lobe of the left lung with impairment of percussion note, rales and bronchial breathing. Pericarditis occurs in patients who have already shown signs of a severe attack and

it seriously worsens the prognosis. Differentiation from heart failure may be difficult but the distinguishing features are italicized in the description which follows.

5. *Heart failure.* This does not generally occur until over *three months* from the onset of the disease and is now very uncommon. There is usually clear evidence of the causative valve disease—commonly mitral reflux with or without association aortic reflux. There is often a striking and unexpected fall of *temperature, white cell count and ESR to normal* with the onset of heart failure, which is also marked by pallor, breathlessness, vomiting, liver enlargement and oedema, together with a raised venous pressure. There may be *small bilateral pleural effusions* and if serial X-ray films have been taken, the increase of heart size will be seen to have been more gradual than in pericardial effusion.

6. *Other signs of carditis.* It has also been suggested that there is tachycardia out of proportion to fever when carditis is present. If however, an increase of twenty beats per minute is allowed for every degree Centigrade of elevation of temperature, a disproportionate increase is rarely found, if causes such as mitral reflux, pericarditis, or heart failure are excluded. Acute dilatation of the heart does not occur unless serious valve lesions have caused heart failure, and then the enlargement is gradual rather than acute.

Chorea

The onset may be marked by emotional lability with abrupt alternations between laughter and tears. There are involuntary movements of muscle groups of the face, a limb, or one side of the body, the movements being infinitely varied and not repetitive as in a habit spasm or tic. They can best be demonstrated by asking the patient to hold the arms and hands outstretched with the tongue protruded and the eyes closed. It will be seen that the affected parts fail to maintain this posture steadily and the hypotonia produces a curious dinner fork deformity at the affected wrist. It may also cause waxing and waning of the grip and a pendular knee jerk. If the involuntary movements are extremely frequent and widespread there may be hyperpyrexia.

Sub-cutaneous nodules

These develop two or three weeks after the onset of a *severe* attack but since the disease has become milder they have become extremely uncommon. Characteristically they occur where the skin moves over bony prominences, along the shins, over the knuckles of the hands, the occipital region and elbows.

Erythema marginatum

This rash is pathognomonic of the rheumatic state but does not necessarily indicate that the disease is active. It consists of red areas which are neither raised nor irritant, and tend to fade in the centre to leave a wavy, spreading border. It occurs on the trunk and limbs but the face is spared.

Other mainfestations

Sometimes the onset of the disease or the early stages of it may be marked by acute abdominal pain and acute appendicitis may be closely simulated.

Differential diagnosis

1. *Cases presenting only with malaise or fever,*

In such cases the diagnosis can only be tentative but is strongly suggested if the AST and ESR are persistently raised and no other cause for the symptoms is found. Cardiographic abnormalities are strongly suggestive but uncommon.

2. *Cases with suspected carditis*

If a diastolic murmur or pericarditis is present the diagnosis is easy. Systolic murmurs occurring in the course of other fevers are distinguished by their softness, early or mid-systolic timing, and poor localisation in the sternal region.

3. *Cases with polyarthritis*

Serum sickness is distinguished by the history and often the occurrence of a raised multiform rash which may be irritant. In Still's disease the small joints of the hands are often affected and the joint pain is more persistent.

4. *Chorea*

Habit spasms or tics are easily distinguished by the endless repetition of the same movement.

Prognosis

The severity of rheumatic fever has been progressively diminishing over the last twenty-five years independently of treatment. The immediate mortality is now probably under 1 per cent. Formerly about twenty per cent of cases died of the disease in the ten years following the attack but this number is now very much smaller. In the past, about fifty per cent of children and twenty per cent of adults suffered from carditis during the course of their disease and at least two-thirds of those who did so were left with permanent valve damage, but these proportions have now dropped by at least 50 per cent.

Treatment

The patient must be kept at rest in bed during the acute phase of the disease; the heart work is least and the patient most comfortable in the semi-recumbent position. Gradual resumption of physical activity is allowed when it becomes difficult to keep the child in bed because he feels well and when the E.S.R. has fallen towards normal.

Penicillin is given in doses of 0.5 to 1.0 mega units daily for ten to fourteen days to clear the throat of haemolytic streptococci. Sodium salicylate in doses of 120 mg/kg/day reducing after three days to 60 mg/kg/day, dramatically relieves joint pains, suppresses fever and reduces the sedimentation rate. It may possibly diminish heart damage by reducing the tachycardia and therefore the cardiac output, but this has not been conclusively proved. If the patient does not respond to this treatment, prednisolone, in a dose of 40 to 60 mg daily according to the weight of the child, is given for three weeks, and then gradually tapered off over a period of eight weeks. The usual side-effects of prednisolone are a hazard, and relapse is more liable to occur on stopping it than on discontinuing salicylates, but in some cases it is invaluable.

Prophylaxis

Penicillin V 125 mg b.d. should be given to all cases until the age of twenty or until five years after the last attack whichever is longer. Alternatively, if the parents or patients are thought unlikely to persevere with daily tablets, the patient should be seen monthly and given 1.2 mega units of Benzathine Penicillin intra-muscularly.

FURTHER READING

Treatment of rheumatic fever in children (1965) Joint report of M.R.C. and American Heart Association. *British Medical Journal*, **2**, 607.

Wilson, M.G. (1940) *Studies in Epidemiology Manifestations Diagnosis and Treatment of Rheumatic Fever*. London: Commonwealth Fund.

Wilson, M.G. (1962) Life history of systolic murmur in rheumatic heart disease. *Progress in Cardiovascular Disease*, **5**, 145.

14. Diseases of the Heart Valves

Mitral stenosis

Morbid anatomy

Mitral stenosis is almost invariably due to rheumatic fever. Narrowing of the valve first occurs by fusion of the cusps at the points of insertion of the shortest chordae tendineae. Over the years a slowly progressive narrowing follows owing to the deposition of platelets and fibrin. Elevation of the left atrial, pulmonary venous and pulmonary capillary pressures is followed by interstitial fibrosis of the lungs and thickening of the alveolar walls, so that the lungs become abnormally stiff. Small haemorrhages may occur into the alveolar walls and decomposition of the haemoglobin to haemosiderin causes brown induration of the lungs. There is medial hypertrophy and intimal fibrosis of the small pulmonary arteries and this may extend to the arterioles. The main pulmonary arteries may also show atheroma associated with pulmonary hypertension which causes right ventricular and right atrial hypertrophy. Finally the persistently raised right heart pressures cause chronic passive congestion of the liver and cardiac cirrhosis.

Haemodynamics

Narrowing of the mitral valve leads to elevation of the left atrial pressure. At first this occurs only during atrial systole; there is exaggeration of the 'a' wave and there is a presystolic pressure gradient between the atrium and the ventricle. If the narrowing increases there is a pressure gradient throughout diastole; the pulmonary venous and pulmonary capillary pressure rise causing vascular engorgement and increased stiffness of the lung. At the same time the pulmonary artery pressure rises passively to maintain the usual pressure difference between the pulmonary artery and the pulmonary veins and ensure a normal blood flow. In the early stages the mean left atrial pressure may be raised to 15 or 20 mmHg but as the stenosis becomes more severe, it may rise to 30 or even 40 mmHg when it will exceed the colloid osmotic pressure of the plasma so that pulmonary oedema results. At these levels, through a mechanism not fully understood, vasoconstriction of the pulmonary arterioles occurs; this predominantly involves the lower lobes so that there is a reversal of the usual distribution of pulmonary blood flow which is normally greater in the lower than in the upper zones. This arteriolar narrowing implies a diminution of the pulmonary vascular bed and is probably responsible for the low cardiac output; the pulmonary artery pressure may rise to as much as 70–100 mmHg with a pulmonary vascular resistance exceeding 9 units.

Clinical features

Women are affected four times as often as men. A history of rheumatic fever is obtained in only about two-thirds of cases and in the remainder the acute attack presumably escaped clinical recognition. There is usually a latent interval of about twenty years between the last attack of rheumatic fever and the development of symptoms. These usually run a course lasting about seven to ten years although recently it appears to have grown longer.

Dyspnoea. This occurs when narrowing of the valve has caused an appreciable elevation of left atrial pressure, with increased turgidity and stiffness of the lungs. Usually breathlessness on effort comes first and later orthopnoea, but sometimes paroxysmal nocturnal dyspnoea is the presenting feature. In the severest form there is pulmonary oedema. This is particularly liable to occur when the cardiac output is increased by emotion, sexual intercourse, infections or pregnancy. There is sudden intense breathlessness, usually in bed at night, followed by the expectoration of pink frothy sputum. Later in the course of the disease, although the left atrial pressure remains high, pulmonary oedema is prevented by the occurrence of alveolar thickening and fibrosis.

Haemoptysis. Sometimes a profuse haemoptysis is the first symptom of the disease. It is due to rupture of a pulmonary vein consequent on the raised pulmonary venous pressure.

Although 500 ml or more of blood may be coughed up, the condition is never fatal, ceases spontaneously, and leaves the patient without symptoms. It is not an indication for surgical treatment. Later in the course of the disease haemoptysis may be associated with pleurisy due to a pulmonary infarct, or may occur as staining of the sputum following an attack of bronchitis or paroxysmal nocturnal dyspnoea. The frothy bloodstained sputum of pulmonary oedema has already been mentioned.

Winter bronchitis. Raised pulmonary venous pressure exaggerates the bronchial congestion and exessive secretion of mucus produced by a cold atmosphere. Bacterial infection is then apt to occur and the characteristic features of acute bronchitis results.

Systemic emboli. These are derived from thrombi which form in the left atrium and especially in its appendage when the blood flow is slowed. They are therefore particularly likely to develop when the cardiac output falls as a result of uncontrolled atrial fibrillation, but may also occur with sinus rhythm. In the first ten days or so following their formation the thrombi are soft and pieces may break off and pass to any part of the body. Hemiplegia, renal infarction or gangrene of the limbs may result.

Angina. This occurs only when severe pulmonary hypertension limits the cardiac output and prevents its normal increase on exercise. As a result the heart work is increased because of the raised pulmonary vascular resistance but the coronary blood flow cannot increase proportionately and pain results.

The facies. If the cardiac output is low, peripheral vasoconstriction in the skin leads to pallor, with areas of capillary vaso-dilatation in which the blood is stagnant and therefore blue. This particularly occurs over the cheeks producing a malar flush.

The arterial pulse. The volume of the pulse is reduced in proportion to the severity of the stenosis, unless there are complicating factors causing vaso-dilatation and increased cardiac output such as pregnancy, infections, hyperthyroidism and so forth. If there is atrial fibrillation the pulse is perpetually irregular in force and frequency.

The jugular venous pressure and pulse. This is normal in uncomplicated cases but if there is severe pulmonary hypertension the 'a' waves are exaggerated and if there is heart failure, the mean pressure is raised. Atrial fibrillation causes absence of the 'a' wave and a poor 'x' descent, with a systolic expansion of the pulse which resembles that of tricuspid reflux but is smaller in amplitude.

The heart. Right ventricular hypertrophy due to pulmonary hypertension leads to a diffuse apical impulse with a tapping quality due to the palpable vibrations of the loud first heart sound. It may also cause a thrust in the parasternal region and pulsation of the pulmonary artery may be felt at the second left space in cases with severe pulmonary hypertension.

In the early stages the acceleration of blood flow produced by atrial contraction in presystole produces a pressure gradient at that time and corresponding murmur. The intra-atrial pressure is high and the intra-ventricular pressure has to rise higher than usual to close the mitral valve, which is thickened. Both these factors tend to produce an unusually loud sound. The result is a crescendo murmur leading up to an abrupt snapping first heart sound. Following the second heart sound there is a delay while the intra-ventricular pressure falls to equal the intra-atrial pressure and then the thickened mitral valve opens with an audible snap about 0.12 seconds after the second heart sound in mild cases. The snap is immediately followed by a murmur as blood flows through the stenotic valve. This dies away quite quickly if the stenosis is mild, but persists quietly throughout diastole if the stenosis is severe. The duration of the murmur is therefore a guide to the severity of stenosis (Fig. 14.1). The delayed diastolic murmur has a low-pitched rumbling quality best heard with a bell chest piece with the patient in the left lateral position. It is usually localised to a small area of the chest wall.

The cardiogram

All cases of more than moderate severity show broadening of the P wave which may measure 0.11 sec or more, with exaggeration of the notch. This is best seen in leads 1 and V6. There may be right axis deviation and if there is severe pulmonary hypertension the precordial leads may show right ventricular hypertrophy (p. 90).

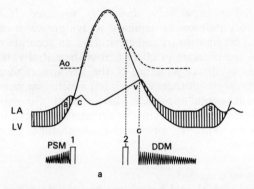

Fig. 14.1 The phonocardiogram of mitral stenosis with the pressure pulses of aorta (Ao), left atrium (LA), left ventricle (LV). A presystolic murmur (PSM) accompanies the presystolic pressure gradient between the left atrium and left ventricle. There is no systolic murmur; the second sound coincides with the aortic dicrotic notch as usual, and when the LV pressure has fallen 0.06–0.10 sec later to equal the LA pressure the opening snap of the mitral valve occurs (C) followed by a delayed diastolic murmur (DDM). Note that the murmur cannot begin immediately after the second sound but is *delayed* until the LV pressure reaches the LA pressure. The murmur persists as long as there is a gradient between the LA and LV. It may cease in mid-diastole and begin again during atrial contraction in presystole. In mild cases it may be present only in presystole while in severe cases it may persist throughout diastole as shown.

Radiology

In the earlier stages the sole abnormality may be selective enlargement of the left atrium seen in the right oblique view and its appendage seen in the postero-anterior view below the pulmonary artery arc (Fig. 4.3 p. 57). The aortic knob is characteristically small unless there is a complicating aortic valve lesion. If there is appreciable pulmonary hypertension, the pulmonary artery and its main branches may be enlarged while the basal sub-divisions are conspicuously narrowed and the upper lobe veins are enlarged. There may be horizontal lines in the costophrenic angles due to lymphatic congestion resulting from the raised left atrial pressure.

Cardiac catheterization

Right heart catheterization is occasionally needed to assess the severity of the disease if the symptoms are equivocal or if associated tricuspid valve disease is suspected. If however, satisfactory pulmonary capillary wedge pressures cannot be obtained by right heart catheterization an accurate measurement of the pressure gradient across the mitral valve can be obtained by direct puncture of the left atrium through the suprasternal notch together with left ventricular puncture, or by the trans-septal approach. Measurement of the pulmonary artery pressure by percutaneous catheterization can be repeated annually to provide an objective assessment of the course of the disease.

Differential diagnosis

Special care should be taken when the diagnosis depends upon a single physical sign, namely a presystolic murmur. This may be simulated by the abrupt first sound in hyperthyroidism or tachycardia resulting from any other cause. In atrial septal defect the first sound may be similar and the diagnosis may be still further confused by the presence of a delayed diastolic murmur, due to the increased flow through the tricupsid valve, which may extend as far as the apex owing to rotation of the heart. However, the correct diagnosis is clearly suggested by the wide splitting of the second heart sound and partial or complete right bundle branch block in the cardiogram together with characteristic radiological features. In cases of mitral stenosis with heart failure or pulmonary hypertension, the characteristic murmur may be absent owing to the low cardiac output and then almost any other form of heart disease may be diagnosed in error. However, an opening snap is commonly present and the radiological appearances are characteristic.

Complications

Atrial fibrillation. This occurs with increasing frequency with age and is almost invariable over the age of forty if the stenosis is well developed.

Sub-acute bacterial endocarditis is relatively infrequent in mitral stenosis and occurs more often in mild mitral reflux.

Congestive heart failure. This is the usual termination of the disease if death is not caused by pulmonary or systemic embolism.

Prognosis

The average life expectation from the onset of symptoms was about seven years but may now be longer.

Treatment

All patients should be given antibiotic prophylaxis for dental extractions, beginning on the day of the extraction and continuing for 5 days to prevent bacterial endocarditis. Atrial fibrillation is treated with digitalis in the usual way and any patient with an uncontrolled tachycardia, due to this or other dysrhythmia, should be given heparin at once followed by a long-acting anticoagulant until the tachycardia is controlled. Anti-coagulants are continued for life in all patients with atrial fibrillation as this substantially reduces the risk of a systemic embolus. Mitral valvotomy should be advised for all patients whose dyspnoea has reached Grade IIa and for those who have suffered from embolism or pulmonary oedema. Heavy calcification of the valve does not preclude a successful operation although it increases the risk and often reduces the benefits obtained. The same is true of advanced age, although patients in their seventh and eighth decades have been operated upon successfully. In such cases and in others in whom the valve is thought to be extremely fibrotic and immobile because the first sound is quiet and the opening snap absent, valve replacement may be found to be necessary and facilities for cardio-pulmonary by-pass should be available at the time of exploration.

Advanced age is no bar to operation, patients in their eighth decade having been operated on successfully, but it increases the risk and diminishes the benefits. However in young patients under the age of twenty-five operation should be deferred as long as possible to avoid re-activation or recurrence of rheumatic fever and premature re-stenosis of the valve.

Mitral reflux

Pathology

There are various causes of mitral reflux but the commonest cause of *severe* reflux is rheumatic fever. The lesion occurs twice as often in men as in women and represents the effect of a more severe attack than that which produces mitral stenosis. It may occur during the period of activity of the disease when the mitral valve ring dilates and the cusps are unable to close the enlarged orifice. After the inflammatory process has subsided a slow fibrosis of the cusps occurs over a period of years so that although the valve ring may return to normal the shrunken cusps are now too small to close the normal sized orifice. In addition fibrosis of the chordae tendineae and papillary muscles interferes with the valve mechanism so that the cusps cannot move back into the closed position during ventricular systole. Finally they may calcify forming a rigid orifice.

Other causes of organic mitral reflux include bacterial endocarditis, myxomatous degeneration (floppy valve) and mitral valvotomy. It can also be produced by other disorders involving the papillary muscles including congenital abnormalities, cardiac infarction, fibro-elastosis, endomyocardial fibrosis and cardiomyopathy.

Functional mitral reflux occurs in conditions causing left ventricular dilatation, namely the later stages of hypertensive heart disease and aortic valve lesions, particularly aortic reflux. Many of these varieties are described subsequently under the heading 'Non-rheumatic mitral reflux' (p. 220).

Haemodynamics

In mild cases the reflux of blood from the left ventricle to the left atrium occurs only in the latter half of systole, when the maximum left ventricular pressure has developed and reversal of the normal direction of flow can occur. If, however, the valves are seriously leaky, reflux takes place almost as soon as the left ventricular pressure begins to rise and lasts throughout systole and even a little after aortic valve closure (Fig. 14.2). There is an abnormal rise of the left atrial pressure, especially in late systole, producing a tall V wave, but its magnitude depends upon the size of the left atrium and the elasticity of its walls. Immediately the mitral valve opens, the left atrial pressure drops almost to zero and equals the left ventricular diastolic pressure. It follows that although the *mean* left atrial pressure is somewhat raised by the high v wave in systole, it is not as high as in mitral stenosis in which the

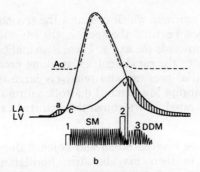

Fig. 14.2 The phonocardiogram of dominant mitral reflux with left ventricular (LV) and left atrial (LA) pressure pulses. The first sound is quiet and a pressure gradient develops between LA and LV immediately afterwards and lasts until just after the second sound. The murmur (SM) is therefore pansystolic and may obscure the second sound. As there is mild stenosis a small gradient develops just after the LA and LV pressures equalize at the peak of the V wave. The resulting delayed diastolic murmur is loud at its onset, may obscure the 3rd sound and dies away quickly.

pressure is raised throughout the cardiac cycle. Consequently the effect on pulmonary venous, capillary and arterial pressures is not as great as in that condition and right ventricular hypertrophy is less marked. The volume work of the left atrium and ventricle however, is increased by the amount of regurgitated blood and there is consequent dilatation and hypertrophy of both these chambers. Ultimately the cardiac output falls and the renal blood flow is reduced. This seems to cause salt and water retention and the syndrome of congestive failure. In contrast to mitral stenosis, pulmonary hypertension is not an essential intermediate stage in this sequence.

Clinical features

If the lesion is moderate or severe there is undue fatigue on effort owing to diminished cardiac output. In mild cases the only sign is a rather high-pitched, late systolic murmur at the apex. In more severe cases the pulse is small in volume and may tend to collapse in late systole, when reflux is maximal. The apex beat is displaced to the left and is hyperdynamic owing to the large stroke volume. The first sound is quiet or absent and there is a harsh, high-pitched or blowing pan-systolic murmur which obscures the second sound. The murmur is best heard at the apex, in the left lateral position, and extends towards the axilla. There is an audible third heart sound owing to the rapid ventricular filling produced by the raised left atrial pressure and relatively large mitral orifice, and a short abrupt low-pitched diastolic murmur may follow owing to the rapid flow through the distorted valve.

The cardiogram

The P waves may be broad and notched due to left atrial enlargement or there may be atrial fibrillation. The QRS voltage is increased due to left ventricular hypertrophy but the T waves are usually upright.

Radiology

There is enlargement of the left atrium and ventricle and calcification of the valve may be seen.

Complications

Embolism is less frequent than in mitral stenosis but endocarditis is commoner, especially in mild cases.

Prognosis

Fatigue occurs early in the course of the disease, but once heart failure has occurred, death usually follows in two or three years.

Treatment

Mild cases due to chronic rheumatic disease may require no treatment apart from careful prophylaxis against bacterial endocarditis. When there are serious symptoms, digitalis and diuretics may relieve them to some extent, but surgical treatment, with the insertion of a prosthesis, offers the only prospect of lasting benefit. When mitral reflux is secondary to another lesion treatment is directed to the underlying cause.

Pregnancy and rheumatic heart disease

The risks and severity of complications produced by pregnancy in patients with rheumatic heart disease has lessened considerably in recent years, probably owing both to a diminished severity of rheumatic heart disease and better supervision in the ante-natal period. Mitral valve disease is the lesion most frequently encountered and disease of the other valves rarely causes any difficulties. Patients with grade 1 or 2A dyspnoea can be allowed to undertake pregnancy without a prior valvotomy though it is probably wisest for such patients to restrict their family to two children. If the degree of breathlessness is greater than this the patient should probably undergo a preliminary mitral valvotomy providing the valve is suitable. The decision between medical and surgical management must be made before the 16th week. After this the risks of surgery progressively increase.

The patient must be carefully supervised throughout pregnancy, three monthly at first, monthly after the sixth month, and weekly during the last month. She should be questioned at each visit for any increase in breathlessness or the development of a cough, which may herald either pulmonary oedema or respiratory infection which sometimes precedes it. Any increase in breathlessness should be treated in hospital with rest and diuretics, and provided the status quo is regained, the pregnancy can be allowed to continue though increased periods of rest may be necessary. Respiratory infection should be treated promptly and vigorously with antibiotics. If the patient does not respond to these measures a valvotomy can be undertaken, provided the valve is suitable, without any added risk to the mother and little risk to the fetus, but is rarely necessary.

Pulmonary oedema

This is the most lethal complication of mitral valve disease during pregnancy. It may occur at any time, though the risk of it gradually increases throughout pregnancy until term and it may even occur during the puerperium. It sometimes occurs without warning in a patient who has been totally free of breathlessness or any symptoms referable to her mitral valve. Occasionally it is precipitated by a respiratory infection or a dysrhythmia but it frequently occurs without evident cause. Treatment with Morphine or Heroin together with an antiemetic, intravenous Frusemide and oxygen should be prompt and vigorous. Digoxin or Aminophyline may also be used and the application of tourniquets at about 50 mmHg for periods of ten to fifteen minutes to three limbs in turn may help to tide the patient over the crisis. After recovery mitral valvotomy should usually be advised without delay to prevent a recurrence.

Contraception and sterilization

Patients with serious heart disease especially rheumatic valve lesions will often be advised to restrict their families to two children. There is no doubt that contraception by 'the pill' is the most reliable and convenient method. Certainly some risks are involved including the development of venous thrombosis, the worsening of arterial hypertension, the possible development of pulmonary hypertension and the disadvantage of a gain in weight. However these risks are small and probably less than those involved by an unwanted pregnancy. Sometimes sterilization is indicated in patients with serious heart disease especially for example, those with pulmonary hypertension which constitutes an extremely grave hazard in pregnancy. Of course this should not be undertaken without very careful consideration of all the psychological and other consequences.

Non-rheumatic mitral reflux and Papillary muscle dysfunction

Abnormalities of structure or function of the papillary muscles and chordae tendineae can lead to important disturbances of mitral valve function. The term papillary muscle dysfunction has been used to cover the wide variety of clinical syndromes which may result. It is, however, far from satisfactory because the function of the chordae cannot be dissociated from that of the papillary muscles and the function of both of these structures has to be considered in relation to the valve cusps. For example, chordae which are too long for normal valve cusps may allow reflux, but chordae which are of normal length may also do so if the cusps are unduly voluminous. It is quite clear therefore that the valve mechanism consists of three components, the papillary muscles, chordae and cusps, which should not be considered separately. It is quite inappropriate to speak of a sub-valvar mechanism of mitral reflux and the term 'sub-valvar mitral incompetence' is even worse for it suggests that regurgitation is occurring through an orifice below the valve.

Non-rheumatic mitral reflux, though clumsy, appears to be the only possible alternative, but since the term papillary muscle dysfunction has obtained fairly widespread acceptance it is used as an alternative in the sense indicated in this introduction.

The normal function of papillary muscles and chordae

These structures have a crucial function to perform in maintaining a suitable position of the valve cusps throughout ventricular systole. During the isometric phase of ventricular contraction sufficient tension must be generated in the papillary muscles to prevent prolapse of the cusps upward into the atrium but not so much to pull them down into the ventricle and open the valve. Then, as the ventricular cavity shortens during the ejection phase, the papillary muscles must shorten correspondingly to take up the slack in the chordae and prevent prolapse and regurgitation.

Situated as they are directly under the endocardium, the papillary muscles are as remote as is possible from the coronary blood supply. They are therefore particularly susceptible to ischaemia. Normally the antero-lateral papillary muscle derives its blood supply from the circumflex branch of the left coronary artery but sometimes there is an accessory supply from the anterior descending branch of the left coronary artery. The postero-medial muscle is supplied either from the circumflex branch of the left coronary artery or the posterior descending branch of the right coronary.

Aetiology and pathology

The main causes of non-rheumatic mitral reflux and papillary muscle dysfunction are shown in Table 14.1. Dilatation of the left ventricular cavity alters the line of pull of the muscles which then tend to hold the valve open during ventricular systole. Such dilatation is particularly prone to occur in aortic reflux. Mitral reflux which develops in this way may be so great as to dominate the clinical picture. Any other cause of left ventricular failure and dilatation, will act similarly. The papillary muscles may be affected selectively by ischaemia or as part of a cardiac infarction or ventricular aneurysm. Atrophic shrinkage of the papillary muscles is common in the elderly who often have a noisy murmur but only slight mitral reflux. Atrophy also occurs in cachectic conditions. Congenital abnormalities are probably fairly common but the lack of morbid anatomical studies makes it difficult to be sure just how often these are responsible for mild degrees of mitral reflux. Certainly however, this can be due to abnormalities of length and origin of the chordae or muscles. In some cases the abnormalities are familial and the clinical picture is then fairly characteristic and is described below. Finally dysfunction of the mechanism may be caused by rupture of the muscles or chordae either spontaneously or following bacterial endocarditis. The remaining possibilities shown in the Table are rather uncommon.

Table 14.1 Causes of non-rheumatic mitral reflux and papillary muscle dysfunction

1. Ventricular dilatation
   Aortic reflux
   L.V. failure

2. Ischaemia
   Localised ischaemia of papillary muscle
   Infarct. Aneurysm.
   Fibrosis

3. Atrophy
   Senile
   Cachexia

4. Congenital anomalies

5. Rupture

6. Endocardial disease
   Endocarditis
   Fibro-elastosis
   Endomyocardial fibrosis

7. Myocardial disease
   Infiltration
   Cardiomyopathy

8. Myxomatous degeneration of the cusps ('Floppy valve')

Haemodynamics

In mild cases the haemodynamics are little altered and may indeed be entirely normal. However, the acute development of mitral reflux causes an extreme elevation of left atrial pressure and pulmonary venous pressure leading to pulmonary oedema. Pulmonary vaso-constriction may result with extreme pulmonary hypertension. The pulmonary artery pressure in such cases is usually well over 60 mm Hg and the pulmonary vascular resistance considerably over nine units. In such cases there is both left and right ventricular hypertrophy.

Clinical features

A wide range of clinical syndromes occurs in this disorder, separable with some overlapping into five main groups.

1. *Asymptomatic non-familial cases.* These patients are discovered on routine examination to have a late systolic murmur as an isolated abnormality (Fig. 2.11). There are no relevant symptoms. X-ray of the chest is normal and there is no enlargement of the left atrium. Proof of the diagnosis has been obtained in some cases by cine-angiography which shows slight mitral reflux confined to the latter half of systole. A few cases in this group show flattened or inverted T waves in leads 2, 3 and AVF and this links them with the next group.

2. *Ischaemic fibrosis or infarction confined to the papillary muscles.* These patients do not invariably give a history of ischaemic cardiac pain and when they do, it sometimes has atypical features. Occasionally however the patient describes typical central chest pain lasting for half an hour or so, without however any of the severe symptoms of cardiac infarction. Sometimes there is transient slight breathlessness on effort. The only abnormal sign in these cases is a late systolic murmur. It seems that the infarcted or fibrotic papillary muscle can hold the mitral valve closed during the early part of systole but cannot shorten sufficiently during the ejection period to prevent regurgitation in the latter half of systole.

X-ray of the chest may show a normal sized heart or there may be slight cardiac enlargement. The cardiogram often shows flattening or inversion of the T waves in leads 2, 3 and AVF, sometimes also in V5 and 6.

3. *Cardiac infarction involving the papillary muscles.* (sometimes with ventricular aneurysm). These patients may present with a characteristic history of cardiac infarction, but this is

not invariable and pain may be atypical or even absent. In such cases the patient may present with acute breathlessness due to pulmonary oedema or breathlessness on effort. There is severe interference with mitral valve function and usually the infarcted papillary muscles fail to hold the valve shut throughout systole so that a pan-systolic murmur results. The patient presents signs of severe acute mitral reflux with high left atrial pressures, pulmonary oedema and pulmonary hypertension. There is a small-volume sharp-rising pulse. The jugular venous pressure is considerably raised and 'a' waves are prominent. Sinus rhythm is the rule. There is evidence of over-activity of both ventricles and commonly there is tachycardia with gallop rhythm and some peripheral oedema. There may be rales over the lungs.

X-ray of the chest shows considerable cardiac enlargement involving both right and left-sided chambers. The pulmonary artery is enlarged as are its main branches but the peripheral branches may be attenuated. The left atrium is not enlarged. The cardiogram usually shows a widespread infarct, sometimes with persistent S–T elevation indicating a cardiac aneurysm.

4. *Rupture of chordae tendineae*. Rupture of the chordae may occur spontaneously in apparently normal subjects or in patients known to have a systolic murmur presumably indicating a congenital mitral valve abnormality. It may also complicate sub-acute bacterial endocarditis. In some patients there is a history of sudden severe chest pain on unaccustomed effort. In others, however, there is no such history and the presentation is with sudden breathlessness on effort or in bed at night, or with congestive heart failure. The physical signs resemble those of Group 3 but the murmur is not always pan-systolic. The timing depends not only upon the function of the papillary muscles and chordae but also upon the degree of ventricular dilatation. Quite often regurgitation is confined to mid-systole and the murmur is maximal at that time resembling the murmur of aortic stenosis (Fig. 14.3). Moreover, if the posterior cusp prolapses, the regurgitant jet may be directed over the anterior cusp towards the root of the aorta so that the murmur radiates to the base of the heart and even into the neck completing the resemblance to the murmur of aortic stenosis. There is however, little difficulty

in differentiating this condition, for in rupture of the chordae the mid-systolic murmur is accompanied by a small volume sharp-rising arterial pulse instead of the slow-rising pulse of aortic stenosis. If the patient survives, signs of pulmonary hypertension develop.

5. *Congenital and familial abnormalities of the chordae tendineae.* A few of these patients rather surprisingly present with chest pain which does not usually have the typical characteristics of ischaemic cardiac pain. It may be felt in the centre of the chest but is often stabbing in quality and unrelated to effort. In many patients there are no symptoms whatsoever and the murmur is discovered on routine examination. As a rule there is but one physical sign, namely a mid-systolic click followed by a murmur which continues to the second heart sound (Fig. 2.11). The cardiogram is usually normal but occasionally shows the pattern described in groups 1 and 2. X-ray of the chest shows no abnormalities but in patients submitted to cineangiography prolapse of the posterior cusp of the mitral valve with late systolic mitral regurgitation has been demonstrated. Some of these patients die suddenly and all are unduly liable to bacterial endocarditis.

Differential diagnosis

In cases with a late-systolic murmur, whether or not this is preceded by a mid-systolic click, the diagnosis presents little difficulty although it may be hard to be sure whether the aetiology is congenital or ischaemic. In patients with a mid-systolic murmur, differentiation from aortic stenosis is easily made by noting the volume and rate of rise of the arterial pulse, as already mentioned, Hypertrophic obstructive cardiomyopathy, in which mitral reflux often occurs, is difficult to differentiate and requires special investigation.

Cineangiography is the most reliable method of establishing the diagnosis for it is usually possible to demonstrate prolapse of a cusp if this is the correct diagnosis. Moreover, it will then be seen that the ventricular cavity is large in contrast to the small deformed cavity of obstructive cardiomyopathy.

Rheumatic mitral reflux is suggested by a pan-systolic murmur, an opening snap, atrial fibrillation, enlargement of the atrium and calcification of the valve.

Prognosis and treatment

This largely depends upon the severity of the mitral reflux. If this is mild, the patient has a nearly normal expectation of life but is liable to the risk of sub-acute bacterial endocarditis and a very few patients die suddenly and inexplicably.

Acute mitral reflux due to rupture of the chordeae or papillary muscles may be rapidly fatal, but many patients respond remarkably to medical treatment with Digoxin and diuretics. If they respond only partially or not at all, they can be dramatically helped by replacement of their mitral valve with a prosthesis.

Mitral stenosis with reflux

Pathology

This lesion is always the result of rheumatic fever and the valve mechanism is more seriously damaged than in pure mitral stenosis. Males are affected more often than females and the cusps and chordae tendineae are fibrotic and shrunken and may be heavily calcified. The orifice usually measures between 1.5 and 2 centimetres in diameter.

Haemodynamics

The features of both mitral stenosis and reflux are combined. The mean left atrial pressure is greatly raised, often with a very large 'V' wave and there is a considerable pressure gradient between the left atrium and ventricle. The pulmonary artery pressure and pulmonary vascular resistance are usually higher than in uncomplicated mitral stenosis so that there is right and left ventricular hypertrophy and ultimately congestive failure.

Clinical features

The symptoms are similar to those in mitral stenosis but may be more severe and occur earlier. The physical signs of stenosis and reflux are combined in varying proportions. If reflux is slight, a pan-systolic murmur alone is added to the signs of mitral stenosis. If it is more severe it may be possible to detect both right and left ventricular hypertrophy and the first sound and opening snap may be inaudible. The reflux produces a high atrial pressure at the end of systole but as obstruction is not severe the diastolic murmur is loud and brief in the first part of diastole and may be preceded by an audible third heart sound (Fig. 14.2, p. 217).

Radiology

Left ventricular dilatation produces a larger heart shadow than occurs in uncomplicated mitral stenosis and calcium is more often seen in the valve.

Angiocardiography

Although it is usually possible to decide on clinical grounds whether serious reflux is present in a case of mitral stenosis, there are occasional cases in which this is difficult and in these cine-angiocardiography is valuable. Contrast material is injected into the left ventricle by retrograde catheterization and the amount of reflux to the left atrium may be directly observed.

Prognosis

The prognosis is intermediate between that of mitral stenosis and mitral reflux.

Treatment

If the reflux is slight the patient is treated as for mitral stenosis. All others are treated as though reflux were the dominant lesion.

Aortic stenosis

Aetiology and pathology

The aetiology of aortic stenosis may be rheumatic, senile or congenital. In rheumatic cases there is adhesion at the commissures and the cusps are fibrotic, shrunken, sometimes calcified and often leaky. In senile cases the cusps are grossly distorted by masses of calcium and their mobility thereby grossly reduced. In congenital cases the valve is often bicuspid and becomes heavily calcified in adult life. In all types males are affected twice as often as females.

Haemodynamics

If the valve area is reduced below 1 sq cm a considerable pressure difference develops across it during systole (Fig. 14.3). The left ventricular systolic pressure is considerably elevated and there is concentric left ventricular hypertrophy. The cardiac output may be low. The distensibility (compliance) of the hypertrophied muscle of the left ventricle is less than normal and a raised left atrial pressure is needed to fill it. The pulmonary venous pressure is correspondingly elevated. Eventually left ventricular dilatation occurs and the elevated pulmonary venous pressure leads to pulmonary oedema. The coronary blood flow is reduced by two mechanisms. The narrow jet emerging from the stenotic valve tends to produce a suction effect on the coronary orifices (Venturi effect) in systole,. while in diastole blood flow is reduced because of the lowered cardiac output. The combination of reduced coronary flow and increased cardiac work results in angina pectoris.

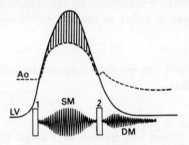

Fig. 14.3 Diagram of the phonocardiogram, left ventricular and aortic pressure pulses in aortic valve disease. Following the first heart sound (1) there is relative quiet while the left ventricular pressure rises to equal the aortic pressure. The murmur (SM) due to ejection then begins, reaches a peak with maximum gradient and flow in mid-systole and then diminishes as ejection declines and ceases before the second sound. (2) *Immediately* following this a gradient develops between the aorta and left ventricle so that the murmur due to an aortic valve leak begins *immediately* after the second sound and may become a little louder before dying away in diastole.

Clinical features

Symptoms are usually absent for as much as twenty to fifty years although a few congenital cases may die suddenly in childhood. The first symptoms may be effort syncope which may be due to transient ventricular fibrillation or to a sudden fall of peripheral resistance and blood pressure. Other early symptoms may be angina of effort or dyspnoea on effort or in bed.

On examination both the arterial pulse and cardiac impulse are found to be slow-rising. A mid-systolic murmur, often with a thrill is usually found at the second right interspace and is transmitted to the neck. Sometimes it may be best heard in the parasternal region or at the cardiac apex and may even be found solely in the latter position (Fig. 14.3). Opening of the valve may produce an ejection click if the cusps are mobile and not calcified. This is most often found in young patients and suggests that the condition is congenital in origin. The blood pressure is usually normal or low but hypertension can co-exist if the stenosis is not extreme.

Radiology

There is post-stenotic dilatation of the ascending aorta and a small aortic knuckle. Calcium may be seen in the valve and if dilatation has followed concentric hypertrophy, enlargement of the heart is also visible.

The cardiogram

This is a more sensitive indicator of concentric left ventricular hypertrophy, and increased voltage, especially in V5 and 6, together with S–T depression and T wave inversion indicate severe obstruction (Fig. 6.15 & 6.16). As usual, *absence* of the characteristic signs is unhelpful and does not deny serious obstruction.

Complications

Bacterial endocarditis occurs occasionally and partial or complete heart block may result from extension of the calcifying process into the adjacent Bundle of His.

Prognosis

If there are no symptoms and the murmur is the only physical sign the patient may survive twenty to fifty years. If left ventricular hypertrophy or a slow-rising pulse is detectable, the expectation of life is probably between ten and twenty years. If syncope, angina or heart failure are present most patients die within two to three years.

Treatment

Surgical treatment by valve replacement offers the only hope of relief of the obstruction and should be offered to all patients with syncope, angina, nocturnal dyspnoea or heart failure. The mortality of the operation at the present time is about five to fifteen per cent, depending on the patient's age, the severity of the cardiographic and radiological features and the co-existence of coronary disease. The more favourable these factors are, the better the operative mortality becomes, but so also does the natural prognosis, and the decision to operate in the absence of the above ominous symptoms is a difficult one.

Aortic reflux

Aetiology and pathology

Aortic reflux may be due to rheumatism, syphilis, athero-sclerosis, bacterial endocarditis or hypertension. It may also be part of the disease of connective tissue in rheumatoid arthritis or ankylosing spondylitis. It may be congenital in origin due to a bicuspid valve, Marfan's syndrome; or as-sociated with a ventricular septal defect or coarctation. In rheumatic and rheumatoid cases there is fibrosis, shrinkage and distortion of the cusps causing reflux but as the commis-sures are also adherent some associated stenosis is common. In syphilis there is widening of the commissures and dilatation of the aorta and aortic valve ring so that stenosis never occurs. In severe hypertension, dilatation of the aorta may lead to slight aortic valve reflux but the cusps are usually normal and there is no stenosis.

Haemodynamics

The volume of regurgitated blood increases the diastolic volume of the left ventricle which is therefore dilated and sometimes has a raised diastolic pressure. Some elevation of left atrial pressure consequently follows and both chambers become hypertrophied. The stroke volume of the left ventricle is increased by the amount of the regurgitated blood and the velocity of flow across the aortic valve is consequently very great. This produces a very sharply rising peripheral pulse which is poorly sustained because of the peripheral vaso-dilatation. The latter seems to be an appropriate circulatory adjustment, for it lowers the peripheral resistance and thus encourages forward flow of blood to compensate for the regurgitation.

Clinical features

Symptoms occur relatively late in the natural history of the disease and the patients may present with nocturnal or effort dyspnoea. Anginal pain may result from the increased heart work, together with poor coronary filling, due to the low diastolic blood pressure. Anginal pain due to aortic incompetence is particularly liable to occur at rest in the recumbent position and may last for hours. On examination there is exaggerated arterial pulsation in the neck and upper extremities (Corrigan's sign), and the pulses are quick-rising ('water-hammer') (Fig. 2.1). Pulsation may be felt in the forearms, and capillary pulsation may be seen as alternate reddening and blanching of the nail beds even without the application of pressure to the nails. The cardiac impulse is hyperdynamic and displaced to the left. An 'immediate' diastolic murmur is usually best heard at the left sternal border and resembles the sound of a whispered 'R'. It follows *immediately* on the second heart sound and is commonly decrescendo but may be crescendo-decrescendo in quality (Fig. 14.3). In addition there is frequently a mid-systolic murmur in the same position or at the second right space due to the abnormally high velocity of blood flow across a roughened valve. The diagnosis of the presence or absence of associated stenosis depends not upon the murmur or even on a systolic thrill but on the quality of the peripheral pulses and cardiac impulse. It must be remembered that significant stenosis of the valve never occurs in syphilis. In severe cases a pre-systolic or delayed diastolic murmur resembling that of mitral stenosis may be heard at the apex. This is the Austin Flint murmur (p. 44) and may be due to partial closure of the mitral valve by the regurgitant flow from the aortic valve.

Complication

Bacterial endocarditis may occur and heart failure may be precipitated by rupture of a cusp either due to the bacterial infection or simply to the effect of mechanical stress on the diseased valve.

Prognosis

The expectation of life after the onset of symptoms is relatively short and is usually between two and five years.

Treatment

Apart from the palliation offered by digitalis and diuretics the only satisfactory treatment is replacement of the diseased valve, either with a prosthesis or a valve homograft. The mortality of the operation is at present about five to fifteen per cent but the results are usually good, at any rate for the period for which they have been observed. There is a morbidity sometimes associated with prostheses, due to infection and emboli and the development of a leak and this may occur in five to ten per cent of cases.

Tricuspid reflux

Aetiology

Tricuspid reflux may be due to rheumatic diseases of the valve when it is always associated with mitral stenosis and sometimes with aortic valve disease as well. More often however, it is functional and due to dilatation of the right ventricle and tricuspid valve ring. The commonest clinical association is mitral stenosis with pulmonary hypertension and atrial fibrillation, but such dilatation may also occur in heart failure from any cause including cor pulmonale, hypertensive and ischaemic heart disease.

Pathology

In cases due to organic rheumatic disease of the valve, the cusps are fibrosed and distorted and there is some associated stenosis. In functional tricuspid reflux the valve ring is greatly dilated and the cusps, though healthy, are not big enough to close the enlarged orifice. The right atrium and ventricle are both dilated and hypertrophied and there is chronic passive congestion of the liver or even cardiac cirrhosis.

Haemodynamics

As a result of reflux of blood from the right ventricle, there is a systolic rise of pressure in the right atrium which is transmitted to the jugular and hepatic veins and produces a characteristic deformity of the wave form of the jugular venous pulse in cases with atrial fibrillation. The 'a' wave and 'x' descent due respectively to atrial contraction and relaxation, are necessarily absent and instead of the normal systolic collapse ('x') there is systolic expansion (cv) due to the regurgitation, followed by an abrupt descent ('y') due to rapid atrial emptying (Fig. 2.3d). Forward flow from the right ventricle is diminished and pulmonary congestion and pulmonary hypertension previously present may be somewhat relieved when tricuspid reflux develops.

Clinical features

Dyspnoea and orthopnoea due to the causative lesion may be lessened when functional tricuspid reflux develops and orthopnoea may even disappear. In severe cases there may be a brownish pigmentation of the skin, ascites and oedema. If there is atrial fibrillation, a large amplitude systolic expansion is found in the venous pulse and sometimes over the liver. At the lower sternum there is a systolic murmur which may become louder in inspiration, but it is a rather difficult and unreliable sign. However, it may be the only physical sign in cases with sinus rhythm, in which abnormalities of venous or hepatic pulsation are absent or difficult to recognise.

Radiology

The right atrium and superior vena cava may be conspicuously enlarged as well as the right ventricle.

Prognosis

In functional tricuspid reflux, the prognosis depends upon the nature and reversibility of the causative condition. Usually it is a late development and the patient has few years to live. In organic tricuspid disease associated with a mitral lesion the prognosis is often slightly better than with a mitral lesion alone, because the lungs are partially protected from congestion.

Treatment

Apart from digitalis and diuretics treatment is of the underlying or associated conditions. Rarely, replacement of the tricuspid valve by a prosthesis, together with mitral valve replacement, may be required.

Tricuspid stenosis

Aetiology

Tricuspid stenosis is almost invariably rheumatic and associated with mitral disease. Often there is aortic valve disease as well.

Haemodynamics

There is a pressure difference across the tricuspid valve in diastole. In sinus rhythm, this is most marked in presystole when 'a' waves measuring 5 to 15 mmHg are found in the atrial pressure pulse but not in the ventricle. More often atrial fibrillation is present and there is then a pressure gradient throughout diastole ranging from 3 to 10 mmHg.

Pathology

The cusps are fibrotic and shrunken and the commissures adherent so that usually there is a fixed narrowed orifice which is both stenotic and leaky. Since the filling pressures of the right heart are normally lower than those of the left, a valve of 2 cms diameter probably causes as serious obstruction to the circulation as a mitral valve of 1 cm diameter. The right atrium is enlarged and hypertrophied as is the right ventricle due to the associated mitral valve disease. There is usually cardiac cirrhosis of the liver.

Clinical features

Tricuspid stenosis tends to prevent the full development of the symptoms of the associated mitral stenosis owing to the restriction of pulmonary blood flow. The jugular pulse shows an exaggerated 'a' wave if sinus rhythm is present and a raised pressure with a cv wave if there is atrial fibrillation. In the former cases a presystolic murmur is heard at the lower sternum while in the latter the murmur follows shortly after the second sound. In either case it may be accentuated by inspiration.

Radiology

In addition to the features of the associated mitral and aortic disease the right atrium and superior vena cava are conspicuously enlarged.

The cardiogram

In sinus rhythm there are tall pointed P waves due to right atrial enlargement and the P–R interval is often prolonged.

Differential diagnosis

The murmur may be difficult to distinguish from that of the associated mitral disease, and a differentiation has often to be attempted between mitral disease with severe pulmonary hypertension and consequent right heart enlargement with *functional* tricuspid reflux, and *organic* tricuspid disease associated as usual with mitral stenosis. In the latter the signs of tricuspid disease are disproportionate to the severity of the pulmonary hypertension resulting from the mitral disease.

Prognosis and treatment

Patients with rheumatic tricuspid disease invariably have serious mitral disease and often aortic valve disease as well. When tricuspid disease is detected they are usually considerably disabled and can be helped for only a relatively short time (2–3 years) by medical treatment. Appropriate surgical treatment of the mitral and aortic valves has then to be considered along with replacement of the tricuspid valve.

FURTHER READING

Symposium (1974) Cardiological aspects of pregnancy. *Progress in Cardiovascular Disease,* **16**(4).

Reichek, Nathaniel., Shelburne, James C., Perloff, J.K. (1973) Clinical aspects of rheumatic valvular disease. *Progress in Cardiovascular Disease,* **15**, 491.

Kremkau, E. Louise., Gilbertson, P.R. & Bristow, J.D. (1973) Acquired non-rheumatic mitral regurgitation. *Progress in Cardiovascular Disease,* **15**, 403.

15. Hyperkinetic Circulatory States

The cardiac output may be persistently raised in a number of conditions, some of them physiological and some pathological. Physiological causes of a hyperkinetic circulation include warm environment, pregnancy, alcohol and emotion. Pathological causes include anaemia, fever, hyperthyroidism, liver failure, arterio-venous communications, Paget's disease and beri-beri. It is doubtful whether the cardiac output is increased in cor pulmonale apart from infections.

Clinical features

These are similar whatever the cause. The hands are warm and there may be capillary pulsation. There is a large pulse volume and the venous pressure may be slightly or moderately raised. There is a tachycardia ranging between 90 and 120 per minute and the high velocity of blood flow may cause an ejection murmur at the base of the heart. If the cardiac output is greatly and persistently raised, mitral reflux may result from papillary muscle dysfunction (p. 221). Rapid ventricular filling produces an audible third heart sound and there may be oedema. Some of the special features of the various causes of a hyperkinetic circulation are now considered individually.

The heart in pregnancy

Haemodynamics and clinical features

The alterations in the circulation in pregnancy are due to the large blood flow through the placenta amounting to an arterio-venous shunt. The increase of cardiac output begins to be detectable at about six weeks and is considerable at the twelfth week of pregnancy. At that time many of the features mentioned above may be found. The venous pressure may be a little raised, the extremities are warm with capillary pulsation and there is often an ejection systolic murmur and third heart sound. The cardiac output continues to increase throughout pregnancy and reaches a maximum between the 30th and 36th week. Thereafter it diminishes gradually until after delivery when it falls abruptly. Late in pregnancy a systolic murmur from dilated arteries in the breasts may be heard.

Anaemia

Clinical features

The hyperkinetic circulation becomes clinically recognisable when the haemoglobin falls below about fifty per cent, and the signs are marked if levels of thirty to forty per cent have persisted for several weeks. Mitral reflux may result from dilatation of the ventricles, and dysfunction of the papillary muscle, and a loud third heart sound may become prolonged into a short low-pitched mid-diastolic murmur. The pulse pressure is large with a low diastolic pressure and there may be considerable oedema.

X-ray of the chest may demonstrate cardiac enlargement and there may be some pulmonary oedema and basal effusions. The cardiogram shows low voltage and flat T waves if the haemoglobin has fallen as low as thirty to forty per cent. These changes are independent of ischaemic heart disease and disappear when the anaemia is corrected.

Treatment

The circulating blood volume is considerably increased in severe chronic anaemia and transfusion may therefore cause heart failure or pulmonary oedema which may be fatal. Transfusion should be given only if the anaemia is refractory, and then packed cells should be given with great caution. All the clinical radiological and cardiographic features resolve following correction of the anaemia.

Hyperthyroidism

Clinical features

In addition to the signs already described, atrial fibrillation is a characteristic feature and is almost invariable in middle-aged or elderly patients. There is then a characteristic failure of the ventricular rate to slow with adequate digitalis administration, although it usually responds to Lugol's iodine or thyroid suppression with neomercazole or radio-iodine. Heart failure with a high venous pressure and oedema does not occur unless there is associated heart disease.

X-ray examination reveals only slight cardiac enlargement unless there is associated heart disease and the cardiogram shows only sinus tachycardia or uncontrolled atrial fibrillation.

Treatment

Digitalis is given in the usual dosage but not excessively for the heart rate cannot be expected to slow until the hyperthyroidism is controlled. Diuretics may be necessary. If atrial fibrillation persists after cure, electrical defibrillation is appropriate. Beta-blockade is dramatically effective.

16. Bacterial Endocarditis

Aetiology and pathology

The aetiology and pathology of this disease has changed considerably in recent years. Formerly, a few cases were caused by an acute infection with staphylococci or haemolytic streptococci affecting an otherwise normal heart, but a sub-acute infection due to streptococcus viridans was much the commonest variety. It affected hearts with congenital or rheumatic lesions and especially those in which a narrow, powerful jet of blood traumatised the endocardial surface. Thus, it was particularly likely to occur in the pulmonary artery adjacent to a patent ductus or on the right ventricular side of a small ventricular septal defect. Among acquired lesions, those with a narrow powerful jet included mild aortic reflux or severe aortic stenosis, or mild mitral reflux, in which a narrow jet impinged on the atrium above. The disease was common in the younger age groups. In recent years however, this pattern of disease has changed in two important respects. It much more often affects the elderly, and the maximum incidence is now in the fifth decade; also it is frequently due to unusual organisms. Occurring in elderly subjects, the under-lying heart lesion is likely to be atheromatous or calcific aortic valve disease which may be quite slight in degree, or mild mitral reflux. Quite often however, a normal valve is affected. Acute infections due to staphylococcus pyogenes are still sometimes seen, but infection with a wide variety of unusual organisms, including streptococcus faecalis, non-haemolytic streptococci, staphylococcus albus as well as aureus, brucella, rickettsial and fungus infections especially candida are common. In the past the usual source of infection was a tooth socket, but now, in elderly subjects, the organisms may frequently come from the gall-bladder, colon, or urogenital tract, especially following operations, and also following childbirth. Infection is now quite frequently seen on prosthetic valves.

Bacteria and fibrin aggregate to form vegetations on the affécted valve or congenital defect. They are large and exuberant in acute cases in which necrosis and perforation of the cusp may occur but smaller in the sub-acute variety in which perforation is less common. Infected emboli may occur in the systemic circulation if the vegetations are on the mitral or aortic valves or on a coarctation and result in septic infarcts in the kidneys, brain, myocardium or lungs. Infected pulmonary infarcts occur if a ventricular septal defect or patent ductus is involved. Streptococcal infection may also cause a concomitant acute or sub-acute nephritis.

Clinical features

In acute cases the patient is obviously seriously ill and has a high fluctuating fever, but in sub-acute cases the onset is insidious with lassitude, weakness, weight loss and low-grade fever. However, some patients, especially the elderly, are afebrile throughout the illness and simply complain of muscular pains, sweating, with palpitations and weight loss, and sometimes symptoms due to a cerebral embolus. In a 'classical' case due to streptococcus viridans in younger subjects the following characteristic clinical picture may be seen. The patients is pale as a result of normochromic anaemia and there may be generalized café-au-lait pigmentation of the skin. Clubbing of the fingers may be seen to develop, first as a reddening and shininess of the skin at the base of the nail and then as an obliteration of the normal obtuse angle between the nail and the skin. There may also be 'splinter' haemorrhages in the finger nails which produce black lines about 1 to 2 mm long in the long axis of the nail. They may be seen in normal subjects but if they are numerous they are probably abnormal. Petechial haemorrhages may be seen in the skin and if they occur in the ocular fundi they may show pale centres. They are probably due to capillary damage indirectly caused by the infection rather than emboli. Red cells in the urine are however, due to micro-emboli in the kidney, and there may be gross haematuria if there is an associated glomerulo-nephritis or a large infarct. Tender nodules in the finger pads or the palms of the hands (Osler's nodes) may be an allergic tissue response rather than embolic in nature. Emboli may also result in large tender lumps in the muscles or the 'silent' disappearance of a peripheral pulse. In a suspected case, the pulsations of all accessible peripheral arteries should be noted when the patient is first seen and the examination repeated daily.

There is usually sinus tachycardia and often slight elevation of the venous pressure. The murmurs appropriate to the underlying congenital or acquired valve disease are found and these may change strikingly during the course of observation if destruction of the valve or chordae tendineae occurs. Thus an aortic diastolic murmur may suddenly acquire a loud whining quality or an apical systolic murmur may become harsh and musical. In such cases there is abrupt worsening of the patient's condition, sometimes with the development of pulmonary oedema or congestive heart failure.

The spleen may be found to be slightly enlarged but since it is soft it may be difficult to feel. The white cell count is raised in acute cases but may be normal or even low in the sub-acute variety. The sedimentation rate is frequently raised. If the infection is not controlled the patient progressively deteriorates and dies in congestive failure.

However, it must be emphasised that this 'typical' picture is no longer common, and the disease is well advanced if all these features are present. The condition should be suspected in any obscure illness in which there is a trivial heart lesion or if there is a slight unexplained fever in the puerperium or in an elderly person following an operation on the gall-bladder, colon or urinary bladder. It must also be considered following the insertion of a heart valve prosthesis if there is a low grade fever, microscopic haematuria, unexplained refractory anaemia and the expected haemodynamic improvement does not occur. The diagnosis is supported if an unexpected murmur develops or if an embolus occurs. These features can however occur in the absence of infection and as the infecting organism is often an unusual one, or even a 'normal commensal' such as a diphtheroid, the diagnosis may be very difficult.

Diagnosis

In the presence of the fully developed clinical picture the diagnosis should be obvious even if the blood cultures are apparently sterile. Nevertheless in these and in more obscure cases both aerobic and anaerobic cultures must be made and kept for several weeks if necessary, to establish the diagnosis, and to determine the sensitivity of the organisms to antibiotics. It may be necessary to begin treatment empirically while awaiting the results.

Differential diagnosis

The condition must be differentiated from other obscure fevers occurring in patients with organic heart disease, and distinction from a recurrence of rheumatic fever may be difficult. Elevation of ESR and anti-streptolysin titre (AST), and the development of heart murmurs, are common to both conditions. However, pericarditis and arthropathy are commoner in rheumatic fever and subcutaneous nodules are characteristic but are now very rare. In difficult cases a therapeutic trial of salicylates, steroids or antibiotics may be needed. Differentiation is particularly difficult after heart operations, when the post-cardiotomy syndrome and intrathoracic infections have also to be considered.

Complications

Emboli may result in hemiplegia, blindness, haematuria, gangrene of the extremities and an 'acute abdomen' due to intestinal or splenic infarction.

Heart failure is an ominous complication and may result from worsening of the valve lesions, the effects of the infection and micro-abscesses in the myocardium.

Prognosis

The disease was uniformly fatal before the advent of chemotherapy and antibiotics. At the present time there is a very wide range of mortality depending upon the nature of the organism, its sensitivity to antibiotics, the stage at which the disease is diagnosed, the age of the patient and the nature of the lesion on which the infection occurs. The mortality may range from 10 to 80 per cent.

Prophylaxis

All patients with minor valve lesions undergoing dental extractions, childbirth, or operations on the gall bladder, colon, or urinary bladder should be given prophylactic antibiotics. These should begin on the day of the operation so that there is no time for resistant organisms to develop in the operation areas.

Treatment

This may have to be initiated before the result of blood culture is known. Almost invariably a combination of antibiotics will be required, and intramuscular penicillin with streptomycin is probably the best pair to begin with. A start could be made with 10 mega units of penicillin and 1 g of streptomycin daily until the infecting organism is known. Then the choice of antibiotics and the dosage should be determined by the concentration of antibiotics shown in the laboratory to kill a large inoculum of the infecting organism. If there is delay in isolating it and the patient is failing to respond, empirical changes in treatment using different combinations of bactericidal antibiotics may have to be used. No dental treatment should be undertaken during the course of treatment and intravenous drips are avoided if possible for fear of introducing fresh infections. If the infection has occurred on a prosthesis and the patient is failing to respond, removal of the infected valve and tissues and replacement with a new prosthesis may be successful. A ductus can be successfully ligated if antibiotic therapy is failing but a ventricular septal defect should be left alone as further infection may occur following closure with a patch. The duration of treatment poses another problem. If the responsible organism was highly sensitive to antibiotics given in relatively low dosage, it is probable that a four week course would suffice, but 8 weeks would be safer. Infection on prosthetic valves or with unusal or insensitive organisms should be given at least 8–10 weeks treatment.

FURTHER READING

Weinstein, Louis & Rubin, R.H. (1973) Infective endocarditis. *Progress in Cardiovascular Disease,* **16**, 239.

Weinstein, Louis & Schlesinger, J. (1973) Treatment of infective endocarditis. *Progress in Cardiovascular Disease,* **16**, 275.

17. Pericarditis

Aetiology

Pericarditis may be infective due to pyogenic organisms, tuberculosis, Coxsackie or other virus infections, and there is a 'benign' idiopathic variety which may be due to an unidentified virus. Other inflammatory causes are acute rheumatism, rheumatoid arthritis, infective mononucleosis, sarcoidosis, systemic lupus erythematosus and other autoimmune disorders. It may also be caused by trauma from injury or operations on the heart, neoplastic infiltration, cardiac infarction, myxoedema, uraemia, and serum sickness.

Pathology

Fibrinous inflammation with little effusion is particularly apt to occur in virus infections, acute rheumatism, systemic lupus, uraemia and cardiac infarction. Adhesions between the visceral and parietal surfaces occur and when the heart is exposed at autopsy a 'bread and butter' appearance results from separation of the adhesions. In tuberculosis there may be a large effusion which is commonly blood-stained but neoplastic effusions are usually straw-coloured. (The reverse is the case in pleural effusions). In pyogenic cases there is pus in the pericardium and in myxoedema a small serous effusion with a high cholesterol and protein content may be found.

Clinical features

The symptoms and signs of the underlying cause will usually be present. Pain is capricious in its occurrence and may be present or absent whether or not there is effusion. It may be precordial in site, and constant, or it may be brought on by coughing, respiration, movement or recumbency. In other cases it may have a phrenic distribution occurring round the lower ribs and in the region of the clavicles. A large effusion may be associated with breathlessness, but if it has accumulated slowly symptoms may be minimal.

Pericardial friction is usually heard best in the parasternal region. In quality it may be high pitched and scratchy or coarse like the creaking of leather. It is often present both in systole and diastole and may be heard even when there is considerable effusion. When this is the case the pericardium becomes taut and filling of the heart is impaired, especially when the pericardial tension is further increased by inspiration. As a result the venous pressure may rise and the arterial pulse volume diminish in this phase of respiration. This is appropriately called a paradoxical venous pulse since it is the reverse of normal. The term 'pulsus paradoxus' applied to the diminution in arterial pulse volume in inspiration is inappropriate since it is in fact merely an exaggeration of the normal response. The area of cardiac dullness may be increased especially in the second intercostal space. The heart sounds are usually quiet and friction, previously noted, may sometimes be observed to disappear. If the venous pressure is very high there may be hepatic enlargement and oedema. In cases with a considerable effusion there are often signs of a small effusion at the left lung base sometimes with rales at the angle of the scapula. This sign of Ewart was formerly attributed to compression collapse of the left lower lobe.

Radiology

In dry pericarditis there are no abnormal features but if there is considerable effusion the heart shadow may be pear-shaped with acute cardiophrenic angles, loss of contours and a wide pedicle (Fig. 4.6). Often, however, this characteristic shape is not seen, contours may be retained and the appearance may resemble that of cardiac enlargement without effusion. Radioscopy is not as helpful as might be expected. The heart shadow is rather motionless if there is an effusion, but an enlarged heart also moves very little.

The cardiogram

In the acute phase of pericarditis there is S–T elevation affecting all limb leads and sometimes the precordial leads as well. After it has returned to the isoelectric level the T waves may become inverted; with a large effusion the QRS voltage is usually low (Fig. 6.19). After complete recovery the cardiogram returns to normal.

The echocardiogram

Echocardiography may be diagnostic of a pericardial effusion (Fig. 17.1), if it shows an echo-free space between the anterior chest wall and the heart or between the left ventricle posteriorly and the pericardium.

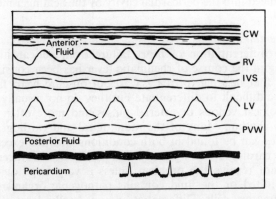

Fig. 17.1 The Echocardiogram in Pericardial Effusion. An echo-free zone produced by the fluid can be seen between the anterior chest wall (CW) and the right ventricle (RV). A similar zone can be seen due to fluid between the posterior ventricular wall (PVW) and the pericardium.

Paracentesis

This may be required for diagnostic reasons, or for tamponade if the pulse is conspicuously small in volume with a systolic blood pressure below 90 mmHg and a venous pressure over 10 cm above S–A. It is best performed at the apex beat, for if the heart is touched, this can readily be detected and no harm is done. It is unlikely that the cavity will be entered and if it is, the puncture seals itself quickly. Alternatively paracentesis can be performed through the xiphisternal notch. This has the advantage that the pleura is not traversed, but the right atrium or ventricle are easily punctured if only a little fluid is present and it may then be doubtful whether there is a heavily blood-stained effusion or a heart chamber has been aspirated. Moreover these chambers seal themselves much less readily than the left ventricle. Whichever method is used a needle of 0.8 mm diameter should be used first and large sizes used only if aspiration is unsuccessful and the presence of pus is strongly suspected. The haemoglobin content of all blood-stained effusions should be estimated. If an extensive exploration is required a catheter can easily be introduced into the pericardial cavity by the Seldinger method (p. 52).

Differential diagnosis

The differentiation of heart failure from pericarditis occurring in the course of rheumatic fever has been considered under that heading (p. 204). Cases of obscure heart failure may be difficult to differentiate but they do not usually have paradoxical venous or arterial pulses and more often have gallop rhythm. Many of the radiological and cardiographic features can be found in both conditions with the exception of the cardiographic signs of acute pericarditis. Paracentesis does not resolve the problem unless a very large quantity is aspirated or the fluid contains pathogenic organisms or inflammatory cells. Differentiation may finally depend upon angiocardiography or the introduction of carbon dioxide into the right atrium through a cardiac catheter and subsequent antero-posterior radiography, with the patient lying on the left side. Pericardial thickening or effusion produces a shadow beyond the right atrial wall. The gas is rapidly absorbed into the blood.

Treatment

Apart from aspiration for tamponade the treatment is that of the underlying condition.

Distinguishing features of some types of pericarditis

Rheumatic pericarditis

There is always evidence of serious carditis with systolic and often diastolic murmurs. Usually there is high fever, pain, breathlessness and pericardial friction which may be creaking in quality. If an effusion is present it is usually small and loculated and does not cause tamponade.

Tuberculous pericarditis

This may occur at any age and affects men more often than women. Fever is variable and may be high or absent. Sometimes a primary focus is discovered.

Benign idiopathic pericarditis

Men are affected three times as often as women and are usually young adults. The condition often follows ten to fourteen days after an upper respiratory infection, and is marked by sudden fever, leucocytosis, pericardial friction and sometimes effusion. The disease runs a course of about six weeks but there may be relapses after intermissions of two to six weeks. Usually recovery is complete but pericardial constriction has been known to follow.

FURTHER READING

Cleland, W., Goodwin, J., McDonald, L., Ross, D. (1968) *Medical and Surgical Cardiology*. London: Blackwell Scientific Publications.

18. Pericardial Constriction

Pathology

The heart is encased in dense fibrous tissue which may be extensively calcified. Sometimes the fibrosis is present in bands occupying the atrio-ventricular sulci. Tuberculosis is the cause of the majority of cases but occasionally 'benign' idiopathic pericarditis, Cocksackie virus infection or rheumatoid arthritis is responsible. However, in many cases the cause cannot be discovered.

Haemodynamics

Filling of the heart is restricted and the venous pressure is therefore high. It falls abruptly but only slightly in early diastole (Y wave) and then filling is suddenly arrested by the inelastic fibrous pericardium, so that the intracardiac and venous pressures then rise abruptly to a plateau which persists throughout the rest of diastole (Fig. 2.3c). The nadir of the Y waves is accompanied by an audible sound due to tensing of the pericardium. Filling of the heart is particularly restricted during inspiration, which increases pericardial tension, and the venous pressure rises and arterial pulse pressure falls in this phase of respiration. The cardiac output is low.

Clinical features

The onset is insidious with fatigue and a variable amount of effort dyspnoea. Sometimes this is quite slight and the clinical presentation is dominated by anasarca with abdominal swelling due to ascites and oedema of the ankles and legs.

On examination the arterial pulse is small and may be 'paradoxical'. The venous pressure is high and the pulse shows an abrupt but shallow Y descent. The blood pressure is usually low and there is atrial fibrillation in about a third of cases.

Properly sustained cardiac pulsations are not felt on the chest but a diastolic shock may be palpable as the sudden inflow in diastole is halted by the taut pericardium and a third sound is almost invariably audible at this point in the cardiac cycle. There may be pronounced ascites, hepatomegaly and oedema.

Radiology

The heart size may be within normal limits or slightly enlarged due to thickening of the pericardium. There is commonly some straightening of the cardiac contours which may assume a triangular shape and calcification may be seen. On radioscopy the heart is conspicuously still or shows only very small amplitude pulsation.

The cardiogram

There is low voltage and flattening or inversion of the T waves (Fig. 6.19). There are often abnormalities of the P wave which may be large or bifid or there may be atrial fibrillation.

Differential diagnosis

Differentiation from a cardiomyopathy may be extremely difficult or even impossible. In such cases, however, the heart is usually larger, there is gallop rhythm rather than the early diastolic sound of constrictive pericarditis and a conspicuous pulsus paradoxus is unusual. The distinction is made easier if the aetiology of the cardiomyopathy is known or if calcium is found in the pericardium. Otherwise the diagnosis may remain in doubt even after cardiac catheterisation and angiocardiography, and an exploratory thoracotomy may have to be performed.

Prognosis

If the clinical picture is fully developed, there is steady deterioration with the development of cardiac cirrhosis of the liver and death follows within a few years.

Treatment

Urgent surgical resection of the pericardium should be advised in all but the mildest cases. The mortality is probably about five per cent and although recovery is sometimes not complete, there is usually considerable improvement. The full benefit of operation may not be apparent for several months after the operation.

FURTHER READING

Cleland, W., Goodwin, J., McDonald, L., Ross, D. (1968) *Medical and Surgical Cardiology*. London: Blackwell, Scientific Publications.

19. Myxoma of the Atria

Pathology

The tumour is usually a rather large, rounded, smooth mass arising by a pedicle from the region of the *fossa ovalis*.

Clinical features

The tumour is commoner in the left atrium where it may obstruct the mitral valve and cause pulmonary oedema, and signs indistinguishable from mitral stenosis. In the right atrium, it may obstruct the tricuspid valve and produce signs of severe congestive heart failure. Both types may be accompanied by fever and greatly raised plasma globulin and ESR.

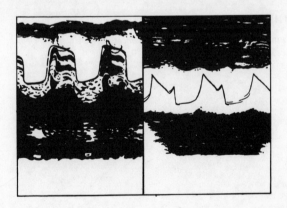

Fig. 19.1 Left. The characteristic appearances in atrial myxoma are shown with multiple echoes beneath the closing slope of the anterior cusp. These are produced by the tumor prolapsing through the mitral valve in diastole. The right-hand panel shows the normal appearances which follows the removal of the tumor. The usual m-shaped configuration produced by the anterior cusp is seen.

Echocardiography

This is usually diagnostic showing multiple echoes behind the trace of the anterior cusp of the mitral valve (Fig. 19.1).

Radiology

The atria are characteristically little enlarged and the tumour may be shown on angiocardiography as a filling defect.

Differential diagnosis

Left atrial tumours must be distinguished from mitral stenosis and other causes of pulmonary hypertension and right atrial tumours from obscure causes of congestive heart failure.

Treatment

The tumour must be removed by open operation with cardiopulmonary by-pass.

FURTHER READING

Goodwin, J.F. (1963) Atrial Myxoma *Lancet,* **1**, 464.

20. Pulmonary Embolism

Pathology

Pulmonary embolism is usually due to a thrombus formed in the iliac or femoral veins becoming detached and passing through the heart to lodge in the pulmonary artery or its branches. The calf veins are a much less common source. Thrombosis may result simply from slowing of the blood flow due to heart failure or to a reduction in blood volume due to haemorrhage or surgical operations. Increased coagulability of the blood is a contributory factor, which may be due to oral contraceptives, accompany neoplastic disease or follow serious trauma or surgical operations. Varicose veins, whether inflamed or not, are not usually the source of emboli. The thrombus probably becomes detached in the first ten days or so following its formation. Later it becomes organised and firmly adherent to the walls of the vein.

The effect of the embolus on the lung and circulation appears to depend chiefly upon its size. A large thrombus becomes lodged either in the main pulmonary artery or in one or both of the main branches and causes obstruction to the right heart with a characteristic clinical picture due to acute right heart failure. Pulmonary infarction does not usually occur in such cases. The reason for this is not altogether clear but it may be that the extremely low pulmonary blood flow due to the obstruction prevents outpouring of red cells into the affected areas so that an infarct does not result. If the embolus is smaller it lodges in the secondary or tertiary branches of the pulmonary vascular tree and then an infarct may occur, usually with a clinical picture resembling pneumonia or 'dry pleurisy', but occasionally without symptoms.

Haemodynamics

Pulmonary infarction produces no significant disturbance of the circulation, but a massive embolism, which obstructs two-thirds of the cross-sectional area of the main pulmonary artery or its two main branches produces an abrupt rise in venous pressure, fall in right ventricular output, and consequently in left ventricular output and blood pressure. The pulmonary artery and right ventricular systolic pressure rises to 40 to 50 mmHg but rarely higher. The right atrial pressure rises to 10 to 30 mmHg.

Clinical features

The condition is common in hospital practice where it may account for as many as three per cent of all deaths. It is well known to occur seven to ten days following surgical operations but is even commoner in medical wards. It may occur in patients suffering from congestive heart failure, neoplastic disease or severe anaemias. It is also particuarly likely to follow seven to ten days after any uncontrolled tachycardia producing a fall in cardiac output. It rarely occurs in ambulant patients suffering from varicose veins but occasionally happens in apparently normal individuals.

As already indicated one of two clinical syndromes may be seen depending upon the size of the embolus. If it is large there is obstruction to right ventricular outflow and acute right ventricular failure, while if it is relatively small there is pulmonary infarction. However, a minority of patients show features of both syndromes. In these cases an inital large embolus may cause obstruction, but subsequent fragmentation of the embolus relieves this and results in multiple pulmonary infarctions. With this proviso the clinical features can be described as two distinct syndromes.

Acute right heart failure due to massive pulmonary embolus

Clinical features

The onset may be marked by sudden intense breathlessness, faintness or syncope. Often there is substernal pain or oppression indistinguishable from ischaemic cardiac pain and suggesting cardiac infarction. This may be due to the abrupt diminution in coronary flow resulting from the low cardiac output together with the increased work of the right ventricle attempting to overcome the obstruction. The patient may be ashen grey or cyanosed, sweaty and breathless. Occasionally symptoms are relatively slight, consisting only of a transient syncope or faintness and yet the cardiogram or the subsequent course may show that a serious embolism has occurred. On examination the venous pressure will be found to be considerably raised, the pulse small and thready and the blood pressure low. There is usually tachycardia and gallop rhythm and a sound resembling pericardial friction may be heard at the base of the heart. This may be due to movement of the dilated pulmonary artery. There may be widespread rales over the lungs due to co-existent pulmonary oedema. The diagnosis is supported if thrombi can be demonstrated in the iliac, femoral or leg veins and methods of detecting them are described later.

The cardiogram

The cardiogram may show various patterns of acute pulmonary hypertension. The electrical axis may shift to the right producing an S wave in lead 1 and a Q wave in lead 3, or there may be right bundle branch block. Sometimes there is S–T depression with T wave inversion in leads 2 and 3 and AVF so that posterior cardiac infarction is simulated. The following chest lead pattern is specific for acute pulmonary hypertension (from any cause) but is seen in only about 30 per cent of cases. There is T wave inversion diminishing in depth from V1 where it is deepest and most long lasting to V4 or 5 where it is shallowest and most transient, together with normal QRS complexes (Fig. 20.1). There may also be transient dysrhythmias.

Radio-active lung scan

This may show perfusion defects but there are many possible causes of this.

Radiology

X-ray of the chest commonly shows no abnormality as infarction does not usually occur.

Pulmonary angiography. A pulmonary angiogram is essential if treatment with Urokinase, Streptokinase or surgical removal of the thrombus is contemplated. A radio-opaque contrast material must be injected through a cardiac catheter placed in the main pulmonary artery under an X-ray image intensifier. The procedure is not without risk and is a rather disturbing

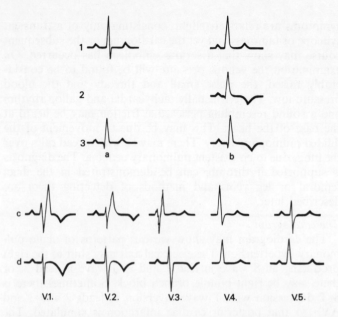

Fig. 20.1 The electrocardiogram may be normal in acute pulmonary embolus or it may show any of the patterns illustrated. The appearance in (a) with an S wave in lead 1 and Q in lead 3 may occur normally but is strongly suggestive if it is seen to develop after a suspicious clinical episode. The same is true of right bundle branch block shown in (c). In (b) the pattern is indistinguishable from an intra-mural inferior infarct. The pattern in (d) with T wave inversion diminishing in depth and persistence from V1 (weeks) to V4 (hours) is diagnostic but less often seen than the other patterns.

one for a seriously ill patient; it does however permit a precise diagnosis and gives accurate information about the extent and localisation of the obstructions.

Haemodynamics. If facilities are available for per-cutaneous catheterization, it is sometimes helpful to measure the pulmonary artery or right ventricular pressure which is moderately elevated with systolic levels of 40 to 60 mmHg. These may be reached in other conditions all of which need to be differentiated including, cardiac infarction, a ruptured papillary muscle and pulmonary oedema. It is not usually elevated in intra-thoracis or intra-abdominal catastrophes.

The detection of venous thrombosis

This is difficult and moreover, most of the clot which has caused the trouble is likely to have travelled to the lungs leaving only a little behind which may be already firmly adherent to the vein wall. Nevertheless every effort should be made to discover its presence as the finding will support the diagnosis and permit well planned prophylaxis to be attempted.

Occasionally there is calf pain and tenderness on direct pressure or on dorsiflexion of the foot with the leg extended and elevated. These signs are, however, unreliable and may be falsely positive or negative and serious emboli more often come from the femoral or iliac veins or their main tributaries. Femoral vein tenderness with slightly raised skin temperature of the affected leg is strongly suggestive of the diagnosis, but only a small proportion of thrombi can be detected in this way. Special techniques have therefore been devised to detect thrombi with greater certainty.

a. *Phlebography*. Radio-opaque material is injected into the dorsal veins of the foot or the saphenous vein at the ankle for demonstration of calf vein thrombosis, or into the femoral veins to delineate the thigh and iliac veins. If the femoral vein cannot be entered an injection can be made through a special needle into the greater trochanter of the femur. These techniques require an X-ray image intensifier to visualise the flow of contrast medium and to time the exposure of X-ray films. The details of technique of injection are crucial, the interpretation of the films may be difficult and requires considerable experience.

b. *The use of radioactive fibrinogen*. An injection of fibrinogen labelled with ^{131}I is selectively taken up by freshly forming thrombus in the leg veins. This is detected by a scintillation counter placed over selected points on each leg. A comparison is made between the counts obtained from corresponding points on each side expressed as a percentage of the count obtained over the heart. An asymmetrically high or rising count over one or more areas indicates accumulation of fibrinogen there and indicates the development of a fresh thrombus. Several doses of radioactive fibrinogen may be needed and the method is unreliable at the proximal part of the thigh, and inapplicable to the pelvic veins where the most dangerous thrombi occur.

c. *The use of ultra-sound.* When a beam of ultra-sound is reflected from a moving object its frequency is altered according to the speed of movement of the object (the Doppler effect). An ultra-sound beam is therefore directed on to the femoral veins and the calves are squeezed to increased the rate of blood flow.. If little or no change in frequency occurs compared with the opposite side an obstruction to flow can be assumed. There is possibly some danger of dislodging clots through squeezing the veins, but the method has the advantage of simplicity.

Differential diagnosis

The cardinal clinical features of massive pulmonary embolism are circulatory collapse with a high venous pressure and low arterial pressure. These features occur in a number of circulatory catastrophes of which the most difficult to differentiate is cardiac infarction. This usually causes chest oppression rather than real breathlessness (unless there is pulmonary oedema) and the venous pressure is rarely very high unless there are complications such as rupture of the interventricular septum or papillary muscles or chordae tendineae. S–T elevation and the pattern of an anterior cardiac infarct point to myocardial infarction but the pattern of posterior infarction also occurs in pulmonary embolism and elevation of transaminases occurs in shock. However, the creatinine phosphokinase, rises early in cardiac infarction and little, if at all, in pulmonary embolus.

Acute pulmonary oedema due to left ventricular failure or mitral valve disease may be surprisingly difficult to differentiate, and it must be remembered that the lungs often become oedematous in massive embolism. Rales and rhonchi may therefore be found in both conditions. They may obscure the murmurs of mitral disease and even suggest acute bronchial asthma.

In paroxysmal tachycardia the patient may have noticed the onset of palpitations before the breathlessness, and a heart rate exceeding 150 per minute, is faster than that commonly found in pulmonary embolism and may respond characteristically to carotid pressure. The cardiogram may show 2:1 A–V block. *It must be remembered that massive pulmonary emolism often occurs in association with any of these conditions.*

Occasionally pericardial effusion has a dramatic onset, with chest oppression, high venous pressure and low arterial pressure; but there is then exaggerated inspiratory diminution of pulse volume (*pulsus paradoxus*) and low voltage with flat T waves in the cardiogram. An abnormal cardiac shadow is helpful if a good chest X-ray can be obtained at the standard distance.

Other causes of sudden circulatory collapse including internal haemorrhage, intra-abdominal or intra-thoracic catastrophes, do not produce a raised venous pressure and in dissecting aneurysm the arterial pressure is often maintained though the venous pressure may rise if there is cardiac ischaemia or rupture into the pericardium.

It will be seen that a wide variety of conditions have to be differentiated and the diagnosis is often made especially difficult by the frequent presence of associated disease.

Finally the diagnosis may be missed altogether if the symptoms consist only of a transient faintness, the nature of which only becomes clear by the occurrence of a second disastrous embolus, the late development of effort dyspnoea or the chance finding of a suggestive cardiographic pattern.

Prognosis
Two thirds of patients survive a first embolus but only one third survive a subsequent one.

Treatment
The patient should be nursed lying flat to safeguard the cerebral circulation and increase venous return, and oxygen should be given. Aminophylline 0.5 g is given intravenously to stimulate respiration and increase the force of cardiac contraction. Cedilanid, or digoxin is given in a dose of 0.5 mg well diluted intravenously and followed by digoxin in maintenance doses. Heroin or pentazocine should be given for pain. An attempt should be made to prevent further emboli with heparin (p. 298). Streptokinase together with corticosteroids to prevent allergic reactions is given parenterally or urokinase can be injected through a cardiac catheter directly into the pulmonary artery to dissolve the thrombi.

If facilities for cardio-pulmonary by-pass are available, surgical removal of the embolus from the main pulmonary artery should be considered but only if the patient's condition, as judged by the respiration, central venous pressure, and blood pressure remains very poor or continues to deteriorate after 2–3 hours. It is especially indicated in patients suffering from a second embolus; or showing widespread occlusions of major branches in the angiogram. In other cases the mortality of operation is usually no less than that of medical treatment, except in specialised centres equipped to establish cardio-pulmonary by-pass with great rapidity.

Pulmonary infarction

Clinical features

The onset is often marked by sudden pleural pain without much breathlessness apart from that due to the pain. There is no syncope or cyanosis but the patient may cough up dark blood or rusty sputum during the following few days. There may be moderate pyrexia up to 38° to 39°C but no disturbance of the circulation. Leg vein thrombosis may be detected by the methods already described. The cardiogram is within normal limits unless there is associated heart disease.

Radiology

The infarct most often appears as a linear shadow or shadows at one or both lung bases with a small pleural effusion in the costophrenic angle. Sometimes there is an irregular shadow or shadows in other parts of the lung, and least often the triangular peripheral shadow, so often described as characteristic is seen.

Differential diagnosis

Pneumonia may be difficult to differentiate but usually the fever and malaise are more conspicuous, and the radiological shadows are more extensive. In both conditions there may be a leucocytosis, but in pneumonia the responsible organism can usually be recovered from the sputum. If the onset is not acute, neoplasms and other causes of lung shadows may have to be differentiated.

Prognosis

All patients recover unless there are subsequent more serious emboli resulting either in acute right heart failure or a syndrome of vaso-occlusive pulmonary hypertension (see p. 266).

Treatment

Pain must be relieved either by pethidine or heroin.

Prophylaxis

The treatment of pulmonary embolism after it has occured is unsatisfactory, and every effort should be made to prevent it. Patients suffering from any of the conditions in which it is a known hazard should be made to wear elastic stockings from the feet to the mid-thighs. These considerably increase the rate of blood flow in the veins and so reduce the risk of thrombosis. They may be as effective as anti-coagulant drugs which can be used in addition, if thought desirable. Heparin in low dosage (3000 units) given twelve hourly subcutaneously considerably reduces the risk of thrombosis and embolism and this should be given to all cases of tachycardia exceeding about 140/min until the dysrhythmia is controlled. Active leg movements or massage and exercises should be encouraged in all patients confined to bed whenever this is practicable. If thrombi have been demonstrated in the major veins, thrombectomy may be considered. Streptokinase can be used to dissolve the clot, but corticosteroids must be given with it to prevent fever or serious allergic reactions. Ligation of the femoral veins or plication of the inferior vena cava have been shown to be both ineffective and dangerous.

FURTHER READING

Symposium (1974) Current problems in pulmonary embolism. *Progress in Cardiovascular Disease*, **17**, nos 3, 4 & 5.

21. Pulmonary Hypertension

Elevation of the pressures in the pulmonary circulation may involve the venous system primarily and the arterial system secondarily or the arterial system may be affected in the first instance by a variety of causes.

The subject may be classified as follows:

1. Pulmonary venous hypertension with passive pulmonary arterial hypertension
2. Pulmonary arterial hypertension
   a. Hyperkinetic
   b. Vaso-occlusive
      i.   vaso-constrictive
      ii. obliterative
      iii. thrombo-embolic

1. Pulmonary venous hypertension with passive pulmonary arterial hypertension

Pathology

The commonest cause of sustained venous hypertension is mitral stenosis; a myxoma of the left atrium can also produce it but is rare. Pulmonary venous hypertension also occurs secondarily to left ventricular hypertrophy and failure of any cause, the commonest being hypertensive heart disease.

Haemodynamics

If the cardiac output remains unchanged with a raised pulmonary venous pressure, the pulmonary arterial pressure must rise correspondingly to maintain the normal pressure difference of about 15 mmHg. This is called passive pulmonary arterial hypertension. If the pulmonary venous pressure is very high, constriction of the pulmonary arterioles may occur and the pulmonary arterial pressure rises disproportionately. The features of this type are described in the section on vaso-occlusive pulmonary arterial hypertension.

Clinical features

The symptoms and signs depend on engorgement of the veins and capillaries resulting in increased stiffness of the lungs. This increases the work of breathing and causes breathlessness on effort, orthopnoea and sometimes paroxysmal nocturnal dyspnoea. In mild cases there are no abnormal physical signs. Rales at the lung bases are due to excess of fluid in the bronchi and not to pulmonary oedema. However, the latter may occur if the pressure is greatly raised and then fine rales or sibillant rhonchi may be found all over the chest..

Radiology

In normal subjects there is a larger blood flow and pressure in the lower, than in the upper lobes of the lung, partly due to the effect of gravity. In mitral stenosis the elevation of the pulmonary venous pressure is greatest in the lower lobes and this apparently leads to selective vasoconstriction of the lower lobe pulmonary artery branches which can be seen to be attenuated. Blood is therefore diverted to the upper lobes, the veins of which can be seen to be distended as they enter the upper parts of the hila. As the venous pressure rises higher, horizontal lines appear in the costophrenic angles due to congested lymphatics. Finally, pulmonary oedema may develop, usually appearing as homogeneous shadows radiating from both hilar regions but sometimes as asymmetrical or patchy shadows.

2. Pulmonary arterial hypertension

a. Hyperkinetic

In this variety the raised pressure results simply from an increased blood flow and there is no increase of vascular resistance. Examples of this variety are seen in congenital malformations with a left-to-right shunt and considerably increased pulmonary blood flow. Since the vascular resistance is not increased it follows that the somewhat raised pulmonary arterial pressure must be transmitted to the pulmonary veins and there is also hyperkinetic pulmonary venous hypertension. This is not described separately as it does not produce a characteristic clinical picture.

Clinical features. The increased vascularity of the lungs causes effort dyspnoea while the excessive blood supply to the bronchi and smaller air passages appears to predispose to repeated respiratory infections especially in young children.

The peripheral pulses are small because of the left-to-right shunt but the heart is hyperkinetic because of the large stroke volume supplied to the lungs. The details of the clinical signs in the heart depend upon the site of the shunt (p. 185-192)

Radiology. The main pulmonary artery and its branches are enlarged and show exaggerated pulsations (hilar dance). The heart is enlarged but its configuration depends upon the site of the shunt.

b. Vaso-occlusive

Patho-physiology

i. *Vaso-constriction.* Severe pulmonary arterial vaso-constriction may occur secondarily to pulmonary venous hypertension in mitral stenosis as already described or in association with congenital heart disease with a shunt (Eisenmenger Syndrome, p. 193). It may also occur in chronic lung disease with anoxia even without prior obliteration of the pulmonary vascular bed or it may occur without evident cause as 'Idiopathic pulmonary arterial hypertension'.

ii. *Obliteration of vascular bed by chest disease.* The arterial and capillary bed is reduced due to extensive pulmonary fibrosis, emphysema, or distortion due to kyphoscoliosis or other chest deformity. Anoxia due to the lung disease has an additive effect causing vaso-constriction.

iii. *Thrombo-embolism of vascular bed.* The pulmonary vascular bed is reduced by repeated emboli to the small arteries or arterioles or failure of lysis of fragments of a large pulmonary embolus.

Clinical features. The cardio-vascular features are shared by all three varieties of the high-resistance type. Functional or anatomical reduction of the pulmonary vascular bed limits the cardiac output and the patient therefore complains of fatigue. Angina may result from the increased cardiac work with a low cardiac output, and effort syncope may occur due to acute right ventricular failure. The low cardiac output results in small peripheral pulses, systemic vaso-constriction with cold extremities and peripheral cyanosis. The right atrial pressure is raised and may be high enough to cause a right-to-left shunt through a patent foramen ovale with the production of central cyanosis. An abnormally powerful right atrial contraction is needed to stretch the hypertrophied right ventricle and as a result there may be exaggerated 'A' waves in the jugular pulse and an audible pre-systolic heart sound. The right ventricle is palpable in the parasternal region or epigastrium and the second heart sound is narrowly split with a loud pulmonary component. There may be an early systolic click and a short mid-systolic murmur as blood is ejected into the dilated pulmonary artery. Later in the course of the disease artial fibrillation may occur with disappearance of the 'a' waves and the appearance of tricuspid reflux with large systolic (cv) venous waves in the neck. The liver is enlarged and there may be liver failure.

The cardiogram. This shows right atrial hypertrophy with tall pointed P waves in leads 2, 3 and V.1., right axis deviation and right ventricular hypertrophy with dominant R waves in lead V.1. and inverted T waves in V.1-3 (Fig. 6.17).

Radiology. The pulmonary artery and its main branches are enlarged but the amplitude of their pulsation is small. The tertiary branches and those in the periphery of the lung fields are attenuated. If mitral stenosis is the cause the attenuation is particulary pronounced in the lower zones. The lungs and heart may show abnormalities due to the underlying disease except in the 'idiopathic' variety.

Differential diagnosis. The above descriptions should enable differentiation of the various types of pulmonary hypertension but differentiation of severe vaso-constrictive pulmonary arterial hypertension which is secondary to pulmonary venous hypertension in mitral stenosis from the primary high-resistance types may be difficult. The signs of mitral stenosis are often obscured if there is severe pulmonary arterial hypertension. The presence of underlying pulmonary venous hypertension, however, is strongly suggested by the presence of orthopnoea and paroxysmal dyspnoea. By contrast when pulmonary arterial hypertension is the primary disorder these features are absent and the clinical picture is marked by fatigue, effort syncope and angina. However, in difficult

CARDIOLOGY FOR STUDENTS

cases it may be necessary to measure the left atrial pressure either indirectly from the pulmonary capillary wedge pressure or by direct puncture.

In some cases, pulmonary stenosis may be surprisingly difficult to differentiate from high-resistance pulmonary arterial hypertension, for both show marked right ventricular hypertrophy with prominent 'A' waves and an enlarged main pulmonary artery. However, in pulmonary stenosis the mid-systolic murmur is much louder, there is often a thrill, splitting of the second heart sound is wider, and the pulmonary component is very quiet. Fallot's Tetralogy may cause, a similar difficulty but the murmur is short and early, and the second heart sound is widely split with a very quiet pulmonary component.

Treatment

This is directed to the underlying cause. Oxygen inhalation temporarily reduces the pressure and long continued anti-coagulation is essential in chronic thrombo-embolic disease. Pregnancy is disastrous in the vaso-occlusive types and must be prevented at all costs.

22. Chronic Cor Pulmonale

Definition

Chronic cor pulmonale is a long-standing disorder of the circulation in which there is episodic or permanent elevation of the pulmonary vascular resistance due to functional or organic disease of the lungs or thoracic cage.

Pathology

The commonest cause of chronic cor pulmonale in the British Isles is chronic bronchitis and emphysema. Other causes include bronchial asthma, neoplastic infiltration of the lung, kyphoscoliosis, fibrosing alveolitis and pulmonary fibrosis due to pneumoconiosis, tuberculosis, sarcoid or other cause. The important factors common to all these conditions are anoxia and diminution of the pulmonary vascular bed. The former causes pulmonary vaso-constriction and the latter also raises the pulmonary vascular resistance. The pulmonary artery pressure is raised at first on effort and later at rest. Other factors, including CO_2 retention, reduced pH, polycythaemia, increased blood volume and cardiac output are probably less important, but all increase the pulmonary artery pressure. Secondary changes occur in the small pulmonary arteries which become narrowed by intimal thickening and medial hypertrophy. Atheroma develops in the large pulmonary arteries and there is hypertrophy and subsequently dilatation of both right ventricle and right atrium. Heart failure eventually results, with the characteristic pathological features in the liver and other organs.

Haemodynamics

In the early stages elevation of the pulmonary vascular resistance may be episodic, especially in the commonest variety due to chronic bronchitis and emphysema. Each attack of bronchitis associated with airway obstruction causes CO_2 retention and some anoxia. The pulmonary vascular resistance rises in the acute attack. In the early stages of the disease it falls to normal with recovery, but if there are repeated attacks, each is liable to leave a residual increment of vascular resistance. The cardiac output has been reported to be greatly raised in cor pulmonale due to chronic bronchitis and emphysema but subsequent investigations have shown the increase to be less than was at first thought. Nevertheless the distribution of the systemic peripheral circulation is unusual, for although the total cardiac output may be scarcely increased the extremities are persistently warm and there is often capillary pulsation.

Clinical features

In cases due to chronic bronchitis and emphysema, men are affected three times as often as women. There is a history of recurrent attacks of winter bronchitis with purulent sputum and sometimes airway obstruction. The length of this history is variable ranging from one to ten years. Sometimes the severity of the cor pulmonale is disproportionate to that of the bronchitis and emphysema, but nearly always the blood gases are abnormal. If sarcoid or neoplasm is the cause, cor pulmonale may develop with remarkable rapidity over the course of a few months. In all cases there is effort dyspnoea but orthopnoea is not a feature.

On examination the patient may be pink and breathless or blue and bloated with congestion of the conjunctivae due to polycythaemia. As usual, cyanosis is best seen in the tongue, but the percentage of arterial desaturation is often less than expected from the depth of cyanosis owing to the presence of polycythaemia (see p. 22).

The earliest sign of cor pulmonale is the development of a pre-systolic heart sound at the lower end of the sternum or over the epigastrium. This is due to the increased force of atrial contraction needed to provide greater diastolic stretch and more powerful contraction of the right ventricle. Later in the disease atrial fibrillation occurs in a proportion of cases and this sign disappears but then tricuspid reflux usually develops. In emphysema right ventricular hypertrophy is detected by palpation upward in the epigastrium and a parasternal thrust is not felt owing to the intervening voluminous lung. The pulmonary component of the second sound is accentuated and splitting may be wide and fixed if there is right bundle branch block. The venous pressure is often elevated and hepatomegaly and oedema may develop. These features may occur even in the absence of an increased pulmonary vascular resistance and the mechanism is not understood. The physical signs of the causative lung disease are usually obvious except in some cases of pulmonary fibrosis or carcinomatosis. In severe cases there may be papilloedema due to raised intracranial pressure with anoxia, and there may be mental confusion or coma due to CO_2 retention. Even in mild cases, the blood gases are almost invariably abnormal, with the PCO_2 above 5kPa and the PO_2 below 13 kPa.

The cardiogram

The heart may be normal in size in the early stages of the disease. Later however, there may be tall pointed P waves in leads 2, 3 and V.1, indicating right atrial hypertrophy (Fig. 6.13). There is sometimes right axis deviation and dominant S waves in leads V.4–6. Lead V.1 may show either an RSR' complex or a dominant R wave (Fig. 6.17). In acute exacerbations there may be T wave inversion deepest in lead V.1 and progressively diminishing towards V.4. These frequently revert, partially or completely, to normal as the exacerbation subsides, as in massive pulmonary embolus (Fig. 20.1).

Radiology

The heart may be normal in size in the early stages of the disease but the main pulmonary artery and main branches are prominent. Later, enlargement of the right ventricle and right atrium is evident. The lungs show evidence of the underlying disease. In bronchitis and emphysema there may be abnormal translucency of the lung bases and the diaphragms may be abnormally flat and low in position.

Diagnosis

The condition has to be differentiated from other causes of right heart enlargement and pulmonary hypertension. These usually lack the characteristic history of chronic bronchitis and emphysema or other underlying lung disease.

In atrial septal defect the heart is more hyperkinetic owing to the large right ventricular output; wide constant splitting of the second heart sound and partial or complete right branch block is invariable. Mitral stenosis with extreme pulmonary hypertension may be difficult to differentiate if the murmurs are absent, but the opening snap is usually audible. Moreover, X-ray reveals left atrial enlargement and often horizontal lines in the costophrenic angles indicating lymphatic congestion due to the raised left atrial pressure. In Eisenmenger's syndrome, primary pulmonary hypertension, and chronic thromboembolic heart disease there is evidence of considerable right ventricular hypertrophy but little or no sign of lung disease. In contrast to cor pulmonale these conditions are commoner in women than in men and the diagnosis depends on the discovery or exclusion of known causes of pulmonary hypertension.

Prognosis

In the earlier stages when pulmonary hypertension completely subsides between attacks of bronchitis, the prognosis largely depends on the prevention of further attacks. If this is successful the patient may live for many years. Once persistent pulmonary hypertension is established, heart failure and death usually follow in a matter of three to five years at the most.

Prophylaxis

This depends entirely upon prevention of recurrent bronchitis, which in turn entails control of air pollution, abstention from tobacco, and prompt control of upper respiratory infections. Cold air is an irritant to the bronchial mucosa and subjects predisposed to bronchitis should avoid outdoor occupations and sleep with their windows closed in the winter. All upper respiratory tract infections should be treated immediately with a seven-day course of antibiotics or alternatively these can be prescribed throughout the winter months.

Treatment

In acute exacerbations the patient requires rest in bed and energetic treatment with antibiotics, antispasmodics, respiratory stimulants and possibly prednisolone. Oxygen must be given with caution because at this stage the respiratory centres are insensitive to carbon dioxide and oxygen-want is their only effective stimulus. A high concentration of oxygen in the inspired air, therefore, leads to hypoventilation and further carbon dioxide retention with the threat of CO_2 narcosis. This can be prevented by the use of Ventimask, which delivers 27 per cent oxygen, and respiratory stimulants such as coramine and aminophylline. Close observation is essential and oxygen therapy is immediately interrupted if respiration slows or becomes shallow; also if there are signs of increasing mental confusion or coma. Digoxin is of a limited value and may be dangerous, but diuretics are given whenever oedema accumulates.

FURTHER READING

Thomas, A.J. (1972) Chronic pulmonary heart disease. *British Heart Journal,* **34**, 7.

Ferrer, M.I. (1965) Disturbances in the circulation in patients with cor pulmonale. *Bulletin of the New York Academy of Medicine,* **41**, 942.

Ferrer, M.I. (1974) Present-day status of cor pulmonale. *American Heart Journal,* **89**(5), 657.

23. Dissecting Aneurysm of the Aorta

Pathology

In this condition the aortic wall is weakened by cystic medial necrosis or by the intrinsic disease of the connective tissue which occurs in Marfan's syndrome. Haemorrhage into the weakened area occurs either from the vasa vasorum or from the lumen of the aorta following rupture of the intima over the weakened area. Three anatomical types have been described as shown in Fig. 23.1. In both of the first two types rupture of the intima occurs a few centimetres above the aortic valve but in the first type the dissection extends both proximally to the aortic valve and distally to involve the great vessels and a variable extent of the descending aorta where a re-entry into the true lumen may occur spontaneously. In this type the dissection may critically narrow the great vessels or lower branches of the aorta resulting in ischaemia of the brain, kidneys or intestines. The spinal arteries may also be involved and dissection of the aorta proximally towards the aortic valve may distort the aortic valve ring and result in aortic reflux. Rupture may occur into the pericardium or into the left pleural cavity or there may be a blood-stained left pleural effusion. In type 2, the dissection is confined to the ascending aorta proximal to the great vessels. In the third type, rupture of the intima occurs just distal to the left sub-clavian artery and involves only the descending aorta. This is the most benign variety, although it too can result in hae-morrhage into the pleura or involvement of the spinal, renal or intestinal vessels.

Clinical features

The onset is usually marked by a sudden violent tearing pain which may be made worse by coughing and deep breathing.

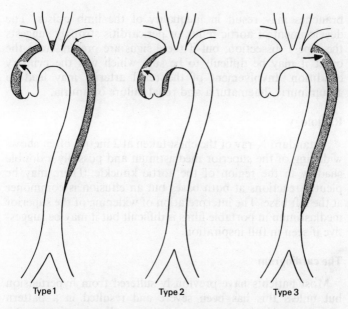

Type 1   Type 2   Type 3

Fig. 23.1 This shows the three main varieties of aortic dissection. In types 1 and 2 the intimal rupture occurs in the ascending aorta within a few centimetres of the aortic valve. In type 1 it extends to involve arch and descending aorta while in type 2 it is confined to the ascending portion. In type 3 the rupture occurs distal to the left subclavian artery and involves the descending aorta.

It is usually much more severe and prolonged than the pain of cardiac infarction. It is felt in the middle of the chest and radiates through to the back. In type 1 lesions, it may be felt severely in the neck and jaw, and if the descending aorta is involved it is also felt in the back, lumbar region and abdomen. In type 3 dissections, the pain may be predominantly epigastric but it may also radiate to the legs, chest or back. There is often breathlessness at the onset and sometimes syncope but although the patient's colour may be ashen, the blood pressure is frequently maintained. There may be mental confusion due to involvement of the carotid vessels and other neurological abnormalities in the trunk and legs may result from involvement of the spinal arteries. Involvement of the major aortic branches may result in inequality of the limb pulses. The development of aortic reflux or pericarditis strongly suggests the type 1 dissection, but if these signs are present from the onset it may be difficult to be sure which was the primary condition. Involvement of the renal arteries may lead to albuminuria, haematuria and renal failure or anuria.

Radiology

A standard X-ray of the chest taken at 2 metres often shows widening of the superior mediastinum and possibly a double shadow in the region of the aortic knuckle. There may be pleural reactions at both bases but an effusion is commoner at the left base. The interpretation of widening of the superior mediastinum in portable films is difficult but it may be suggestive if seen in full inspiration.

The cardiogram

Most patients have previously suffered from hypertension but unless this has been severe and resulted in a pattern of left ventricular hypertrophy the cardiogram is normal. Occasionally the pattern of sub-endocardial ischaemia with ST depression in the chest leads may be seen and in a few cases there may be evidence either of concomitant infarction or pericarditis.

Prognosis

Without treatment three-quarters of the patients die in the first two weeks and the prognosis is especially bad in types 1 and 2. There is also an appreciable late mortality and less than 10 per cent of untreated cases are alive at the end of one year.

Treatment

It has been shown that careful and persistent reduction of the systolic blood pressure to 100 to 140 mmHg for two or three weeks greatly improves the prognosis and enables elective surgery to be undertaken when the tissues have regained some strength through fibrosis and the general condition of the patient has improved. Immediate reduction of the blood pressure is achieved with diazoxide 300 mg in an intravenous bolus followed by increasing oral dosage of propranol beginning with 40 mg 6-hourly. Alternatively methyldopa (Aldomet) 250 to 500 mg in 100 ml of 5 per cent dextrose 6-hourly can be given intravenously until the pressure is controlled and then the same does is given by mouth 8-hourly. Later bendrofluazide (Aprinox) 5 mg daily with potassium supplements can be added to potentiate the other drugs. Sedation with diazepam (valium) is also helpful. Complete bed rest is essential for at least 3 weeks although sometimes this period can be shortened without harmful effect. Unless there is dramatic internal haemorrhage or dangerous ischaemia of the brain or limbs, consideration of surgical treatment is deferred for 6 to 8 weeks. If it is not altogether contra-indicated by associated disease or senility, preliminary aortography is performed to show the site of the tear and the extent of the dissection. Type 1 and 2 lesions require cardio-pulmonary by-pass, while type 3 requires only left heart by-pass. The aorta is transected and the separated layers of its walls sutured together. Continuity can sometimes be re-established by end-to-end anastomosis but more often the insertion of a graft is required.

FURTHER READING

Slater, E.E. & De Sanctis, R.W. (1976) Dissecting aneurysms. *American Journal of Medicine,* **60**, 625.

Wheat, Myron W. Jr. (1973) Treatment of dissecting aneurysms of the aorta. *Progress in Cardiovascular Disease,* **16**, 87.

24. The Cardiomyopathies

Definition

The cardiomyopathies may be defined as a group of diseases affecting the heart muscle either primarily or as a part of a generalised disease involving other parts of the body.

Classification

A. Cardiomyopathies secondary to other diseases
   1. Neurological diseases
      a. Muscular dystrophy
      b. Friedreich's ataxia
      c. Dystrophia myotonica
   2. Metabolic and other diseases
      a. Amyloid disease, Primary or secondary
      b. Systemic lupus erythematosus, polyarteritis, and rheumatoid arthritis
      c. Alcoholism
      d. Beri-Beri
      e. Myxoedema
      f. Haemochromatosis
      g. Glycogen storage disease
      h. Mucopolysaccharide storage disease
      i. Sarcoid
      j. Loeffler's syndrome
      k. Cirrhosis
B. Primary disorders of heart muscle or endocardium
   1. Idiopathic—Hypertrophic—sometimes familial
      a. With variable outflow obstruction
      b. With inflow restriction (Restrictive cardiomyopathy)
   2. Idiopathic cardiomyopathy with congestive failure
   3. Fibro-elastosis.
   4. Endomyocardial fibrosis; a condition confined to natives of certain parts of Africa, characterised by

progressive thickening of the ventricular endocardium often spreading to involve and distort the atrioventricular valves.

Presentation

Although many of these varieties have distinguishing features a detailed description of them is beyond the scope of this book. In general, their clinical presentation takes one of the following three forms:

a. A picture resembling that of aortic stenosis—the hypertrophic obstructive type
b. a picture resembling contrictive pericarditis
c. congestive heart failure.

These three syndromes are described in the following account of the primary cardiomyopathies.

Hypertrophic cardiomyopathy

Pathology

The condition is characterised by hypertrophy of the cardiac muscle without evident cause. The muscle fibres are abnormally short and thick. Sometimes the hypertrophy is markedly asymmetrical and mainly involves the septum but more often it is generalised. It may cause obstruction to outflow of the left ventricle, and in some cases there is also obstruction to outflow of the right ventricle.

Mitral reflux is very often present and is occasionally due to abnormal attachment of the mitral valve, but more often there is no evident primary anatomical cause, and disordered function of the papillary muscles must be assumed.

Haemodynamics

Obstruction by hypertrophied muscle results in the development of a systolic pressure gradient in the outflow tract of the affected ventricle. This occurs in mid-systole as full contraction develops. Consequently the peripheral pulse rises sharply at first but then abruptly falls off as the forward flow is obstructed. A quick-rising small-volume pulse results. The gradient across the obstruction is increased by adrenaline, noradrenaline and isoprenaline and exercise; it is diminished by drugs which block the beta-adrenergic receptors and by rest. As a result the symptoms and signs are characteristically variable.

Clinical features

The condition may be familial and siblings may have died suddenly or be known to have a murmur. The patient may complain of dizziness or syncope especially on effort, angina and fatigue. There may be effort dyspnoea or paroxysmal nocturnal dyspnoea. Sometimes however, symptoms are completely absent and attention is drawn to the condition by the presence of a murmur.

On examination the pulse is characteristically small in volume and quick-rising, although there is a powerful left ventricular impulse and basal mid-systolic murmur. Thus the impulse and murmur suggest aortic stenosis but this is contradicted by the pulse (p. 21). This combination at once suggests the correct diagnosis. Sometimes the cardiac impulse has a double thrust owing to the presence of a palpable atrial contraction. There may also be an apical pan-systolic murmur due to associated mitral reflux. The blood pressure is usually normal but a raised pressure may have been observed in the past leading to the suggestion that the condition is simply one of hypertensive heart disease in which the pressure has fallen but hypertrophy remains. There is insufficient evidence to uphold or refute this theory. In some cases right ventricular involvement may be associated or even dominate the clinical picture, with or without outflow obstruction simulating pulmonary valve stenosis.

The cardiogram

This usually shows evidence of left ventricular hypertrophy with tall voltage and T wave inversions in lead 1 and V.4–6. Sometimes there is left bundle branch block. In cases with obstruction to the right heart there may be right ventricular hypertrophy and in either case there may be evidence of atrial enlargement with tall or broad P waves.

Radiology

The size of the heart shadow is frequently normal as hypertrophy occurs at the expense of the cavity.

Cardiac catheterisation and angiocardiography

Catheterisation of the right or left heart or both is needed to demonstrate the gradient, and selective angiocardiography of the affected ventricle shows an abnormally small cavity with an irregular outline due to encroachment by muscle masses, and especially by the hypertrophied papillary muscles.

Differential diagnosis

Aortic stenosis may be closely simulated but is distinguished by a slow-rising pulse and calcification of the valve. Rheumatic mitral reflux is suggested if there is a delayed diastolic murmur, other valve lesions, calcification of the mitral valve and tall R waves in leads 1, V5 and V6 without S–T depression or T wave inversion. Non-rheumatic mitral reflux (p. 220) may be very difficult to differentiate as papillary muscle dysfunction may occur in both conditions. If however, there is a mid-systolic click, a late systolic murmur and flat or inverted T waves in leads 2, 3 or VF non-rheumatic mitral reflux is easily recognised. Ischaemic heart disease may present difficulties as angina is variable in both conditions and the cardiogram may be similar. However, evidence of concentric left ventricular hypertrophy is lacking, outflow obstruction does not occur and mitral reflux, if present, is usually associated with signs of ventricular aneurysm or flat or inverted T waves in leads 2, 3 and VF. However, in some cases, left ventricular and coronary angiography may be needed to distinguish the two conditions. Neurosis may be suggested by the symptoms of fatigue and faintness but physical signs are absent unless there is coincident disease.

Prognosis

This is uncertain as the condition has only been described comparatively recently. All patients however, are unduly liable to the risk of sudden death but many survive ten years.

Treatment

The obstruction and angina can be diminished or even abolished by beta-adrenergic blocking drugs such as pro-pranolol, but large doses may be needed. Surgical treatment by interruption of masses of obstructing muscle fibres or their complete resection has been practised but results are difficult to assess and medical treatment is now generally preferred.

Restrictive cardiomyopathy

Pathology

The pathology is ill-defined but includes amyloid disease. There is no outflow obstruction.

Haemodynamics

The hypertrophied ventricle is inelastic and resists filling. The venous pressure is therefore high and the cardiac output low as in constrictive pericarditis. The venous pulse shows a pronounced 'Y' dip which however, returns abruptly to a plateau which persists through the rest of diastole (Fig. 2.3c, p. 25).

Clinical features

The clinical picture may be identical in all respects with that of constrictive pericarditis and the only distinguishing feature may be the lack of evidence of pericardial thickening in angiocardiograms. This syndrome is also seen in many of the secondary cardiomyopathies particularly those associated with neurological disorders, amyloid and collagen disease and leukaemic infiltrations.

Treatment

There is no specific treatment unless a primary cause can be found.

Cardiomyopathy with congestive failure

Pathology

The heart is dilated but not appreciably hypertrophied and in some cases there may be no histological abnormality. In others there may be round-cell infiltration. The aetiology is probably varied in this group of cases and may include virus infection, hypersensitivity and metabolic causes.

Clinical features

There is congestive failure without evident cause and cardiac hypertrophy is not detectable. There is usually gallop rhythm and often tricuspid or mitral reflux.

The cardiogram

The cardiogram often shows low voltage with flat or inverted T waves in many leads or left bundle branch block.

Treatment

Digitalis and diuretics are given in the usual way.

FURTHER READING

Goodwin, J.F. (1970) Cardiomyopathies—A decade of study. *Lancet*, **1**, 731.
Goodwin, J.F. & Oakley, C.M. (1972) The cardiomyopathies. *British Heart Journal*, **34**, 545.

25. Resuscitation

Great advances have recently been made in the resuscitation of the apparently dead by the introduction of external cardiac massage and the rediscovery of the value of mouth-to-mouth artificial respiration (Elisha's method—Kings II. 4.34).

Indications

Attempts at resuscitation should be made in all cases of *unexpected* death. This will naturally include cases occurring before, during and after surgery, electrocutions and Adams-Stokes attacks. In addition the procedure will be indicated in many but not all cases of cardiac infarction and pulmonary embolism. In such cases, the physician in charge should say in advance if resuscitation is to be attempted, and indeed this decision should be made with regard to all patients in hospital.

Method

Speed is essential to success and if more than *three minutes* elapse between the cessation of heart action and the institution of effective methods, death is inevitable. The first person on the scene must not leave the patient, but must *shout* for help, and immediately begin resuscitation. The patient is placed either on a bed-board, or on the floor and external cardiac compression is begun. The operator kneels beside the patient, placing one hand over the other on the lower end of the sternum and compressing it rhythmically at a rate of about 60–70 per minute in adults (faster in children) so as to depress it about 4–6 cm. Excessive force must not be used and it is usually possible to avoid the fracture of ribs. The production of a palpable femoral or carotid pulse is the minimum criterion of effective external cardiac massage. The procedure is interrupted every thirty seconds to apply mouth-to-mouth artificial respiration. A handkerchief can be interposed if a Brook airway is not available. During this procedure, the nasopharynx should be cleared of mucus and vomitus, the nostrils of the patient should be pinched, the jaw held forward, and the chest should be seen to rise during inflation. After three or four breaths cardiac massage is resumed and the two procedures continued alternately. When help arrives a Brook airway is inserted or the patient is intubated and continuous ventilation is maintained, either with air or oxygen. If cardiac arrest persists for more than thirty seconds metabolic acidosis develops and should be promptly countered by the intravenous infusion of 50–100 ml of 8.5 per cent sodium bicarbonate. An intravenous drip should be set up and a total dose of about 3mEq/kg body weight may be needed; and one tenth of this can be given every ten minutes. Persistence of ventricular fibrillation is frequently due to acidosis and prompt correction is vital if cardiac action is to be restored. If it does not occur within a few minutes, a cardiogram should be obtained to determine whether there is asystole or ventricular fibrillation. In the former case 4–10 ml of 1/10 000 Adrenaline is injected into the left ventricular cavity through a needle inserted in the region of the cardiac apex and directed towards the posterior aspect of the right shoulder. (Adrenaline may also be helpful in cases of ventricular fibrillation). 5–10 ml of 1 per cent calcium chloride may also be effective in cases of a complete standstill as it increases the contractility of the heart.

If the cardiogram shows ventricular fibrillation d.c. shock is the most effective remedy. The skin is prepared with electrode jelly and one electrode is placed at the second right interspace and the other at the cardiac apex. Shocks are applied at energy levels ranging from 150 to 350 W/s, and the cardiogram is observed after each shock.

If a satisfactory rhythm is not restored the cause may be either inadequate oxygenation or acidosis. The former should be checked by ensuring that the airway is clear and the latter by estimation of the standard bicarbonate, but while the result is awaited, it is usually safe to give a further dose of sodium bicarbonate intravenously. Following d.c. shock arrhythmias are sometimes observed. Ventricular tachycardia is treated with 4–10 ml of 1 per cent lignocaine intravenously and bradycardia by 0.1 mg of isoprenaline. If the cardiographic complexes are of reasonably normal contour on the oscilloscope, massage should nevertheless be continued until a spontaneous peripheral pulse can be felt.

If spontaneous respiration and an effective heart beat do not occur it must be decided whether to persist with resuscitation or not. Persistence is indicated if the condition leading to the arrest would ordinarily have been expected to have a fairly good prognosis and if the start of resuscitative measures was prompt, produced satisfactory oxygenation and a palpable femoral pulse. It should certainly be continued if the pupils have not become widely dilated and if any electrocardiographic activity is visible on the oscilloscope.

Aftercare

The patient should be nursed in a semi-recumbent position, if conscious. Otherwise he must be placed recumbent with the head dependent and turned to one side to facilitate drainage of secretions. Adequate oxygenation must be ensured and intubation or even tracheostomy may be indicated together with the administration of oxygen. The cardiogram must be monitored continuously for dysrhythmias and the blood pressure recorded every quarter of an hour. Acidosis and hypotension may need to be countered with bicarbonate and isoprenaline or the infusion of 5 per cent glucose as described in the section of 'Treatment of cardiac infarction complicated by cardiogenic shock' (p. 173). The venous pressure should be monitored by a polythene catheter inserted into a vein and connected to a saline manometer. The stomach should be aspirated and urine output measured. A careful watch should be kept on the serum electrolytes and blood gases and appropriate adjustments made to maintain normal values. If cerebral oedema is suggested by prolonged unconsciousness with restlessness and signs of raised intra-cranial pressure, surface cooling should be employed and dexamethasone 4–20 mg is given i.m. or intravenously.

FURTHER READING

Rowlands, D.J. (1976) Cardiac arrest. *British Journal of Hospital Medicine*, **16**, 310.

Gilston, A. & Resnekov, L. (1971) *Cardio-respiratory Resuscitation*. London: Heinemann.

26. Anxiety State With Cardiovascular Symptoms

In some subjects the fear of the presence of heart disease or association with relatives or friends who suffer from it may lead the patient to attribute chest pains to heart disease. An anxiety state develops and the symptoms become more obtrusive. In young people, an anxiety state may arise from an initial association of fear with effort, such as fear of drowning when learning to swim or of injury while playing football or rugby. The pounding of the heart, due partly to fear and partly to exertion, may be interpreted as evidence of heart disease and causes further anxiety with worsening of the symptoms. The commonest of these is left infra-mammary pain and this has already been described (p. 16). It is of interest that although the patient may be familiar with the characteristics of angina, either as a result of medical training or observation of his relatives, his own anxiety symptoms are quite different and have the characteristics of psychogenic pain previously described. This is also true if an anxiety state follows cardiac infarction, when the patient may have both typical angina and an anxiety-type pain, each having their own distinguishing features.

Palpitations, perpetual tiredness and inability to undertake physical exertion are other common symptoms. Dizziness may occur on effort or prolonged standing or even when the patient is seated or recumbent. The latter circumstances exclude a primary circulatory disorder. There is often undue breathlessness on effort and the patient may be observed to hyperventilate both on effort and at rest, when respiration may be punctuated by frequent deep sighs.

There are no abnormal physical signs but severe cases may show excessive sweating of the axillae, palms of the hands and feet, but not of the body. The extremities are cold and blue and there may be a slightly raised blood pressure. There is tachycardia, a hyperkinetic cardiac impulse, and often a basal mid-systolic murmur due to the rapid circulation. The cardiogram and X-ray are within normal limits unless there is associated organic disease.

Differential diagnosis

Mitral reflux may be suspected if the patient happens to have an innocent apical systolic murmur and fatigue is the main symptom. However, if symptoms are due to mitral reflux, some cardiac enlargement, especially involving the left atrium is usually found. Atrial septal defect may be suspected because of the basal mid-systolic murmur and a hyperkinetic cardiac impulse but wide splitting of the second sound, partial or complete right bundle branch block and the characteristic radiological appearances are absent.

Mitral or aortic stenosis should cause no difficulty but the severity of the lesion must be carefully assessed to decide whether the symptoms are entirely attributable to it or whether they are partly due to an anxiety state.

Differentiation of ischaemic cardiac pain may be extremely difficult, if it is atypical and especially if it is associated with pain due to an anxiety state. Such an association has already been mentioned (p. 154). A cardiographic effort test may be very valuable in establishing the presence of ischaemic heart disease, but if it is equivocal or negative, and important doubt remains a coronary angiogram may be required, though that too may not always solve the problem.

Hyperthyroidism may be very difficult to differentiate for it is always accompanied by an anxiety state. The hands, however, are usually warm, and sweating involves the whole body. Tremor is fine and not coarse as in anxiety and there may be eye signs and thyroid enlargement. Nevertheless, in difficult cases it may be impossible to exclude hyperthyroidism without recourse to thyroid function studies.

Finally it must be repeated that neurotic symptoms differ sharply from those of organic disease and if the patient's complaints are compatible with the latter they must be provisionally accepted as such, even though the patient also has psycho-neurotic traits. In medical practice the doctor-patient relationship as well as the patients' health are commonly and repeatedly jeopardised by the failure of the doctor to accept the patient's story as true. The history should always be accepted at its face value unless there are *overwhelming* reasons to the contrary. The patient is almost always telling the truth exactly as it appears to him and skilful and intelligent history-taking is often the most important single step the doctor makes in arriving at a correct diagnosis.

A diagnosis of circulatory disturbance due to psychiatric disorders should rest on two points. First, organic disease is absent or insufficient to account for the symptoms: second, the patient has a psychoneurotic personality and adequate grounds for the production of symptoms.

Prognosis

The condition tends to be self-perpetuating and may even become gradually worse over the years as the symptoms produced by each new attempt at physical exertion further alarm the patient.

Treatment

The first essential is a complete clinical investigation so that the patient can be convincingly assured that he has no organic heart disease. If there is associated organic heart disease the problem is more difficult and an attempt must be made to persuade the patient that his symptoms do not arise from it. Next an explanation is given of the mechanism and nature of the symptoms; they are not imaginary but consist of an abnormal awareness of the physiological responses to emotion and effort. Persistent reassurance is needed to persuade the patient to undertake physical effort and to disregard the symptoms. Progressive physical exertion, supervised either by a physiotherapist, school teacher or parents, is needed to restore the patient to normal activity. Despite all these efforts, progress is often very slow and the final result far from satisfactory.

27. Action of Drugs

Adrenaline

Action

Stimulation of alpha and beta-sympathetic receptors causing increased force and rate of the heart beat, coronary vaso-dilatation, skin vaso-constriction and pronounced muscle vaso-dilatation so that there is only a transient rise of blood pressure. It is a broncho-dilator and has many other effects depending on alpha and beta stimulation.

Uses

Motivation of the heart in cardiac arrest due to standstill or to ventricular fibrillation.

Dose

1–5 ml of a 1/10 000 solution intravenously or directly into the ventricular cavities.

Amiloride hydrochloride (Midamor. Combined with Hydro-chlorothiazide as Moduretic)

Action

Causes increased excretion of sodium and chloride and reduced excretion of potassium, by an action on renal tubules.

Uses

Prevention of potassium depletion caused by diuretics in the treatment of oedema.

Dose

10 to 20 mg daily.

Unwanted effects. Dizziness and weakness.

Aminophylline (Cardophylin)

Action

Respiratory and cardiac stimulant.

Uses
Heart Failure. Pulmonary oedema. Cheyne-Stokes Respiration.

Dose
100–300 mg by mouth. Suppositories of 360 mg. 250 mg in 10 ml water slowly i.v.

Unwanted effects. Gastric irritation with nausea and vomiting. Intravenous use has resulted in sudden death and it must be given slowly and cautiously.

Amiodarone

Action
Prolongation of action potential and refractory period.

Uses
Supra-ventricular tachycardias and other dysrhythmias

Dose
Preparations not yet available in British Isles.

Anti-dysrhythmic drugs

Action
Drugs used for the treatment of dysrhythmias or the suppression of premature beats can be roughly classified according to their *predominant* mode of action as follows:

1. Slowing of depolarization
   Lignocaine
   Mexiletine
   Disopyramide
   Quinidine
   Procainamide
   Phenytoin
2. Anti-sympathetic
   Beta-blockers (Propranolol, etc.)
   Bretylium
3. Prolongation of action potential and refractory period.
   Amiodarone
   Sotalol

4. Calcium antagonism
      Verapamil
      Prenylamine

For ventricular tachycardias and ventricular premature beats, group 1 drugs are usually the first choice.

For supra-ventricular tachycardias, drugs in groups 2, 3 or 4 are usually the first choices.

Atropine

Action

Paralyses the para-sympathetic nerve endings resulting in increased heart rate.

Uses

In sinus bradycardia following cardiac infarction, digitalis toxicity and vaso-vagal attacks.

Dose

0.6 mg subcutaneously or well-diluted intravenously

Unwanted effects. Dry mouth, pupillary dilatation and tachycardia.

Bendrofluazide (B.N.F) (Aprinox)

Action

Diuresis is produced by diminished re-absorption of Sodium, Potassium, Chloride and water from the distal tubules of the kidneys. Potassium loss may be considerable and supplements are usually given during the acute phase of the illness. For this reason a combined tablet containing Potassium Chloride is useful to avoid a multiplicity of medications.

The blood pressure is reduced partly through Sodium and Chloride depletion but also through the renin-aldosterone mechanism. This does not become fully effective until about two weeks after the beginning of treatment.

Uses

Treatment of oedema and hypertension.

Dose

2.5 to 10 mg daily

Neo-Naclex K contains 2.5 mg of Bendrofluazide with 630 mg of Potassium Chloride.

Navidrex K contains Cyclopenthiazide 0.25 mg with 600 mg of Potassium Chloride.

Unwanted effects. The most important is Potassium depletion which is particularly liable to occur when dietary intake is poor as in the elderly and in the acute phase of the illness. It also tends to produce hyperglycaemia and glycosuria and may precipitate gout. The serum uric acid should be estimated at the beginning of treatment and Allopurinol given if it is high.

Beta-receptor blocking drugs (Propranolol, oxprenolol, and others)

Action

These drugs combine with the beta-adrenergic receptors thus preventing adrenaline from doing so and at the same time having little or no stimulating (sympathomimetic) effect. The extent of the sympathomimetic effect is variable among the members of the group which have the following *four* main effects in varying degrees:

1. Reduction of the rate and contractility of the heart, with consequent diminution in oxygen demand and relief of angina.

2. Reduction of blood pressure. The mechanism is uncertain as the effect is not adequately explained by 1 and an action on the renin-aldosterone mechanism is unproven.

3. Broncho-constriction through blockade of bronchodilator receptors.

4. Membrane-stabilising effect which tends to suppress premature beats and ectopic rhythms.

Dose

See individual Drugs

Uses

Treatment of angina, hypertension, obstructive cardiomyopathy, and cyanotic attacks of Fallot's Tetralogy. Control of heart rate in hyperthyroidism and of blood pressure during removal of phaeochromocytoma and in dissecting aneurysm.

Unwanted effects. Excessive bradycardia. Also see individual drugs.

Bethanidine (Esbatal)

Action

Blocks adrenergic impulses and thus lowers the blood pressure.

Uses

Treatment of hypertension.

Dose

10 to 100 mg twice daily.

Unwanted effects. Muscular weakness, dizziness, postural hypotension, fluid retention, failure of ejaculation or impotence.

Bretylium (Darenthin)

Action

Blocks sympathetic effects.

Uses

Ventricular-ectopics, tachycardia and fibrillation, and other dysrhythmias.

Dose

100 to 200 mg t.d.s monitoring the blood pressure.

Unwanted effects. Hypotension.

Bumetanide (Burinex)

Action

Similar to Frusemide but possibly more rapid in effect and may produce less Potassium loss.

Uses

Treatment of oedema and heart failure.

Dose

1 to 2 mg mane

Unwanted effects. Potassium depletion.

Clonidine (Catapres)

Action

Reduction of the blood pressure by largely unknown mechanisms. Probably it has an effect on the central nervous system reducing peripheral sympathetic activity.

Uses

Treatment of hypertension.

Dose

0.1 to 0.3 mg three times a day

Unwanted effects. Sedation, drowsiness, salt and water retention.

Digitalis preparations

Digoxin and Lanatoside C. (Cedilanid). There has been a remarkable diminution in the use of digitalis preparations for heart failure in recent years. Since its effectiveness was established by Withering in the 19th century digitalis preparations have been among the most powerful and useful drugs in the treatment of heart failure. The present decline in their popularity is no doubt due to the increased incidence of toxic effects usually resulting from potassium depletion produced by diuretics. The correct approach is to use diuretics and potassium supplements correctly and to control the doses of digitalis preparations with proper care and skill. They should undoubtedly remain the corner-stone of treatment of congestive heart failure and many dysrhythmias.

Only two preparations need be considered. They are, digoxin (Lanoxin) and Lanatoside-C (Cedilanid). The actions of both are similar although Lanatoside is claimed to have a wider margin between the toxic and therapeutic dosages.

Action

Both preparations increase the excitability and contractility of the heart. The resulting increased efficiency reduces the diastolic volume and pressure, diminishes oxygen consumption and slows the rate. Further actions include a reduction in conductivity of the A–V junctional tissues and vagal stimulation producing slowing of the ventricular rate in atrial fibrillation and termination of supraventricular tachycardias.

Uses

Heart failure. Atrial fibrillation and flutter. Supraventricular tachycardia.

Digoxin dose schedules

For average adults

Rapid	*Standard*
1–1.5 mg stat	0.5 mg t.d.s. for 1 day
1.0 mg in 8 hours	0.25 mg q.d.s. for 1 day
0.75 mg after further 8 hours	0.25 mg t.d.s. for 1 day
– 0.25 mg daily or b.d. maintenance	0.25 mg daily or b.d.

Elderly	*Infants*
0.25 mg q.d.s. 1 day	Total dose 0.8 mg/Kg
0.25 mg t.d.s. 1 day	$\frac{1}{2}$ total dose stat, then
0.0625 mg –	$\frac{1}{4}$ total dose in 8 hrs and
0.125 mg daily or b.d.	$\frac{1}{4}$ total dose in 8 hrs
	1/5 of total = daily maintenance

Toxic effects

Toxic effects are particulary likely to occur if there is potassium depletion which occurs with vigorous diuretic therapy, and in the aged whose intake of potassium may be low and whose excretion of digitalis may be slow.

A. *Gastro-intestinal effects.* These are the commonest and include anorexia, nausea and vomiting and occasionally diarrhoea.

B. *Dysrhythmias.* Ventricular premature beats and coupling may occur but the latter is not necessarily a sign of digitalis overdosage. Any dysrhythmia whatever may be due to digoxin overdosage but supraventricular tachycardia with 2 to 1 block is especially common. Ventricular tachycardia and even ventricular fibrillation may also occur. Development of a slow regular nodal rhythm in atrial fibrillation is also characteristic of digitalis overdosage, and all grades of A–V block may develop in sinus rhythm.

C. *Cerebral effects.* Malaise with headaches are common but drowsiness and confusion are rather rare.

D. *Visual disturbances with yellow vision.* These occur occasionally.

Disopyramide (Rythmodan)

Action

Stabilises cell membranes slowing depolarization.

Uses

Ventricular premature beats, ventricular tachycardia and fibrillation also other dysrhythmias.

Dose

100 to 200 mg t.d.s.

Unwanted effects. Nausea, vomiting, malaise, bradycardia, cardiac standstill.

Frusemide (Lasix)

Action

Powerful inhibition of re-absorption of Sodium, Potassium, Chloride and water from the proximal and distal tubules and ascending loop of Henle. It has a rapid action lasting for only about 4 hours.

Uses

Treatment of oedema. (It is not very effective in hypertension)

Dose

Average 40 to 80 mg but 180 mg or more daily can be given. Intravenously 20 to 40 mg. Children 1 to 3 mg per kg daily.

Note: Frusemide is rarely the drug of choice for maintenance therapy for which the Thiazides are usually preferable. In unusual instances the patient may prefer the rapid effect of Frusemide to the slower prolonged effect of the Thiazides which are much more economical.

Glyceryl trinitrate

Action

Glyceryl Trinitrate produces relaxation of smooth muscle and widespread vaso-dilatation resulting in flushing, throbbing headaches and tachycardia with a fall of blood pressure. The relief of angina is probably due to the lowering of peripheral vascular resistance together with increased myocardial blood flow due to dilatation of collateral vessels.

Uses

Relief of angina

Dose

0.3 mg is probably optimal but 0.5 to 1 mg may be given at each dose and repeated as often as necessary with a minimum interval of thirty minutes. The tablets should be dissolved in the mouth because absorption is through the buccal mucous membrane. A sustained release tablet (Sustac) can be swallowed in a dose of 2.6 mg or 6.4 mg.

Heparin

Action

Inhibition of the conversion of prothrombin to thrombin, antagonisation of thromboplastins and inhibition of conversion of fibrinogen to fibrin.

Uses

Prevention of thrombosis.

Dose

15 000 units intravenously every 12 hours. A low dose regime of 3000 units subcutaneously every eight hours has been shown to be effective in preventing venous thrombosis in the legs.

Unwanted effects. Overdosage may cause epistaxis, haematuria, and retro-peritoneal haemorrhage. Dosage can be controlled by estimation of the clotting time which should be maintained at twice normal. If it is excessively prolonged the effect of Heparin can be reversed by intravenous Protamine in 1 per cent solution. If given within 15 minutes of the dose of Heparin, 1 mg of Protamine neutralizes approximately 100 units of Heparin. After a longer time interval less Protamine is needed and not more than 50 mg should be given at any one time.

Isoprenaline (Saventrine = long acting oral preparation)

Action

Isoprenaline is a synthetic analogue of Adrenaline having similar actions but lacking alpha receptor effects. It therefore increases the rate and force of the heart beat with only a slight rise of blood pressure.

Uses

Stimulation of the heart at cardiac operations or cardiac arrest. Used orally in a long-acting form it can be tried for complete A–V block, but doses which increase the rate usually produce intolerable side-effects.

Dose

0.01 to 0.05 mg intravenously or into the heart chambers for cardiac arrest or by intravenous drip of 10 per cent solution at 1 ml per minute. Oral long-acting Isoprenaline 30–120 mg four times a day according to tolerance.

Unwanted effects. Pounding of the heart with throbbing of the head vessels and apprehension.

Lignocaine

Action

Stabilisation of cell membranes, slowing depolarization.

Uses

Ventricular premature beats and ventricular tachycardia and fibrillation.

Dose

1 mg/kg intravenously stat then 1 mg/min infusion.

Toxic effects. Mental confusion and convulsions.

Mexiletine

Action

Stabilisation of cell membranes slowing depolarization.

Uses

Ventricular ectopic beats ventricular tachycardias and fibrillation.

Dose

Intravenously 100 to 200 mg

Orally 400 mg, then 200 to 250 mg eight hourly.

Unwanted effects. Nausea, vomiting, drowsiness, nystagmus, tremor, bradycardia, hypotension.

Oxprenolol (Trasicor)

Action

Similar to Propranolol.

Uses

Treatment of angina, hypertension and dysrhythmias.

Dose

20 to 80 mg or more 3 times a day after a test dose of 20 mg.
Unwanted effects. Similar to Propranolol.

Oxygen

Action

The reduced arterial oxygen tension occuring in heart failure and following cardiac infarction predisposes to serious dysrhythmias. The arterial oxygen tension is frequently reduced in pulmonary hypertension and raising it by oxygen administration may lower the pulmonary vascular resistance. In respiratory failure a low arterial oxygen tension is accompanied by chronic carbon dioxide retention which no longer stimulates the respiratory centre. Lowering the arterial oxygen tension by administration of oxygen may deprive the body of its sole remaining stimulus to respiration. The Co_2 tension rises and may cause narcosis.

Uses

Heart failure, cardiac infarction, pulmonary embolism. High concentrations must not be used in respiratory failure especially when due to chronic bronchitis and emphysema with cor pulmonale.

Administration

The Ventimask is made in four patterns delivering 24 per cent, 28 per cent, 35 per cent and 40 per cent oxygen. The M.C. mask delivers 24 per cent to 29 per cent at one litre/min and 41 per cent to 70 per cent at four litres/min. A high concentration should only be used if it is certain that there is no carbon dioxide retention. If these masks are not well tolerated, 'spectacles' with nasal catheters can be used but these give lower concentrations of oxygen.

Unwanted effects. Carbon dioxide narcosis. Retrolental fibrodysplasia in premature infants treated with concentrations exceeding 50 per cent.

Perhexiline (Pexid)

Action

Reduction of exercise tachycardia. Improvement of left ventricular function with increased stroke work index for a given left ventricular filling pressure. It increases myocardial lactate extraction and oxygen extraction during controlled tachycardia.

Uses

Treatment of angina.

Dose

100 to 200 mg twice daily.

Toxic effects. These are quite common in the early stages of treatment and include dizziness, headaches, nausea and vomiting. Occasionally nervousness, tremors, ataxia, syncope and flushing or sweating. All may be abolished by reduction of dosage. Peripheral neuritis demands withdrawal.

Phenytoin (Epanutin)

Action

Stabilises cell membranes slowing depolarization.

Uses

Ventricular ectopics, ventricular tachycardia and fibrillation, also other dysrhythmias.

Dose

100 mg b.d. or t.d.s.

Unwanted effects. Gastro-intestinal upset, allergic reactions, unsteadiness, blood dyscrasias.

Potassium (Kloref, Slow-K, Sando-K)

Action

Potassium is the dominant intracellular cation and is vital for the normal functioning of all body cells. Potassium depletion is commonly caused by potent diuretics and results in muscular weakness, paraesthesiae and cardiac dysrhythmias with an increased tendency to digitalis toxicity. It should be noted that the serum potassium is a rather poor guide to the body content of potassium which is largely intracellular.

Uses
Correction or prevention of potassium depletion.

Dose
Each tablet of the above preparations contains about 8 m.eq. of potassium; 2 to 8 tablets a day are needed depending on the amount of diuresis. Intravenously the maximum safe dose is 20 m.Eq. per hour.

Unwanted effects. Potassium chloride may cause ulceration of the small bowel but the risk of this is minimised by the use of sustained release tablets. Rapid intravenous infusions may cause the heart to stop in diastole. Contraction can be restored by the intravenous injection of calcium gluconate.

Prenylamine (Synadren 60)

Action
Probably coronary vaso-dilatation and inhibition of uptake and storage of catecholamines in the heart. In contrast to beta-blocking drugs it does not diminish myocardial contractility and so does not cause heart failure and it does not cause bronchial constriction.

Uses
Treatment of angina.

Dose
60 mg 3 to 5 times daily.

Unwanted effects. Nausea, vomiting, diarrhoea, hypotension.

Procainamide

Action
Stabilisation of cell membrane slowing depolarization.

Uses

Prevention and treatment of dysrhythmias especially ventricular ectopics, ventricular tachycardia and fibrillation.

Dose

250 mg 4 to 6 hourly.

Toxic effects. Gastro-intestinal upset. A syndrome resembling systemic lupus erythematosus may follow prolonged administration.

Propanolol

Action

Propanolol is the most widely used of a group of drugs which block beta-adrenergic receptors. They relieve angina by diminishing the oxygen demand of the heart by slowing it and reducing myocardial contractility. They lower the blood pressure by an unknown mechanism. Reduction of contractility does not account for this effect fully and an action on the renin-aldosterone mechanism is unproven. Some of the drugs in the group have a membrane stabilising effect and therefore tend to suppress ventricular premature beats and dysrhythmias.

Uses

Treatment of angina, hypertension and dysrhythmias.

Dose

40 to 360 mg three times daily after a test dose of 20 mg.

Unwanted effects. Excessive bradycardia, depression, lack of energy and occasionally idiosyncrasy with fainting and low blood pressure. Reduction of myocardial contractility may cause heart failure if serious heart disease is present. It may aggravate asthma by blocking broncho-dilator impulses. This tendency may be less pronounced with some members of the group which are more cardio-selective, including Metoprolol (Lopressor and Betaloc) Timolol (Blocadren).

Quinidine (Kinidin durules)

Action

Stabilisation of cell membranes slowing depolarization.

Uses

Ventricular premature beats, tachycardia and fibrillation, also other dysrhythmias.

Dose

As Kinidin durules, 250 to 500 mg 8 hourly.

Unwanted effects. Hypersensitivity causing urticaria, fever, headache, tinnitus and partial deafness. Nausea and vomiting can be caused by overdosage.

Sorbide nitrate

Action

Generalised vaso-dilatation with a fall of blood pressure and flushing. It has a similar but milder effect than glyceryl trinitrate. For relatively rapid action it should be dissolved in the mouth but for prolonged action it can be swallowed.

Uses

Relief of angina.

Dose

5 to 10 mg sublingually; 20 to 100 mg daily in divided doses to be swallowed for prolonged action.

Unwanted effects. headaches, flushing, fainting and methaemaglobinaemia.

Spironolactone (Spironolactone BP, Aldactone)

Action

Spironolactone is a steroid structurally resembling aldosterone and acting as a competitive inhibitor of it. It therefore increases sodium and water excretion by the kidneys and diminishes potassium excretion.

Uses

Potentiation of diuretics and prevention of potassium depletion.

Dose

25 mg 2 to 4 times daily.

Unwanted effects. Headaches, rashes and gynaecomastia.

Streptokinase

Action

Streptokinase is an enzyme activator derived from the growth of haemolytic streptococci. It converts plasminogen present in the human serum to a fibrinolytic substance plasmin. In contrast to Urokinase it can be given systemically and then has a general action throughout the body.

Uses

Lysis of thrombi especially venous thrombi in the legs and pulmonary emboli.

Dose

100 000 to 500 000 units intravenously followed by 200 000 units for four hours and 100 000 units per hour for up to three days in a continuous drip.

Unwanted effects. Streptokinase is antigenic and may cause a serious allergic reaction with high fever. This may be supressed with concomitant treatment with Hydrocortisone and Prednisolone. Haemorrhage may occur from any site and blood coagulation should be estimated and haemorrhages treated with amino-caproic acid.

Urokinase

Action

Urokinase is an enzyme obtained from human urine which converts plasminogen present in human serum to plasmin which is a fibrinolytic substance.

Uses

Lysis of pulmonary emboli.

Dose

200 000 to 300 000 ploug units in saline through a cardiac catheter into the pulmonary artery over a period of two hours.

Unwanted effects. Haemorrhage and fever rarely.

Verapamil (Cordilox)

Action

Interferes with calcium metabolism and shows depolarization.

Uses

Supra-ventricular and other tachycardias.

Dose

40 mg or more 8 hourly.

Unwanted effects. Hypotension, bradycardia, cardiac standstill.

Warfarin sodium

Action

Delays clotting prolonging prothrombin time by inhibiting the formation of Factor *VII* and prothrombin. Prolonged action with half-life of about 48 hours.

Effects persist for 5 days.

Uses

Prevention of venous thrombosis.

Dose

Initial 20–30 mg. Measure prothrombin time in 36 hours, then 3–10 mg daily to maintain prothrombin time 2–2.5 × normal

Action enhanced by: Alcohol, Salicylates, Clofibrate, Butazolidine, Antibiotics, Allopurinol, Steroids.

Action reduced by: Barbiturates.

Unwanted effects. Overdose causes bleeding especially from gums, in skin, from urinary tract and in retroperitoneum.

Toxic effects. Alopecia, Urticaria.

Treatment of overdose. Vit K 5–20 mg i.v. Use minimum dose or there may be difficulty in restoring prothrombin time to therapeutic range. If severe, give fresh plasma.

FURTHER READING

Baller, G.A., Smith, T.W., Abelmann, W.H., Haber, H., Wood, W.B. (1971) Digitalis Toxicity. *New England Journal of Medicine*, **284**, 989.

Fisch, C., Zipes, D.P. & Noble, R.J. (1975) *Digitalis Toxicity: Mechanism and Recognition in Progress in Cardiology* 4. Philadelphia: Lea and Fibiger.

Symposium on Beta-blockade (1976) *Postgraduate Medical Journal*, Supp(**4**), 52.

Martindale's Extra Pharmacopeia (1977)
London: Pharmaceutical Press

Index

A-V block, *See* Atrioventricular block

A-V junctional tissue, 73

A-V node, effect of interruption of conduction at various levels, 121

Accelerated phase high blood pressure,
cardiogram, 134
clinical features, 133
radiology, 135
urine, 135

Acidosis,
contributing to ventricular tachycardia, 115, 116
in ventricular fibrillation, 117

Actin filaments, 1

Acute endocardial ischaemia, cardiography, 96

Acute epicardial ischaemia, cardiography, 95

Acute right heart failure due to pulmonary embolus,
cardiogram, 257
detection of venous thrombosis, 259
differential diagnosis, 260
haemodynamics, 258
prognosis, 261
pulmonary angiography, 257
radio-active lung scan, 257
radiology, 257
treatment, 261

Acyanotic congenital heart disease, studied by angiography, 61

Adrenaline,
influencing heart rate, 2, 3

Albuminuria, and high blood pressure, 136

Aldactone, in congestive heart failure, 13

Aldosterone,
in congestive heart failure, 13
in myocardial disease, 7

Allopurinol, in treatment of high blood pressure, 138

Amiloride hydrochloride, 290

Aminophylline, 290
in treatment of pulmonary oedema, 11

Amiodarone, 291

Amyloid disease, 8

Anacrotic pulse, 21

Anaemia,
clinical features, 237
treatment, 237

Aneurysm, in palpation of the heart, 30

Angina pectoris, in ischaemic heart disease, 151
cardiogram, 153
clinical features, 151
differential diagnosis, 154
anxiety pain, 154
cervical spondylosis, 155
hiatus hernia, 155
indigestion, 154
duration of pain, 152
episodic and linked angina, 156
in mitral stenosis, 211
physical signs, 153
prognosis, 155
quality of pain, 151
relationship of pain to increased heart work, 151
site of pain, 151
treatment, 155

Angiography, 60

Angiotensin, 1, 2, 131

307

Anti-dysrhythmic drugs, 291
Anxiety state with cardiovascular
        symptoms, 287
    differential diagnosis, 288
    prognosis, 289
    treatment, 289
Aorta,
    enlargement of, 58
    in palpation of the heart, 30
Aortic aneurysms, studied by
        angiography, 61
Aortic arch abnormalities, studied
        by angiography, 61
Aortic reflux,
    aetiology and pathology, 230
    clinical features, 231
    complications, 231
    haemodynamics, 230
    in rheumatic fever, 204
    prognosis, 232
    studied by angiography, 204
    treatment, 232
Aortic stenosis,
    aetiology and pathology, 227
    cardiogram, 229
    clinical features, 228
    complications, 229
    haemodynamics, 227
    prognosis, 229
    radiology, 229
    treatment, 229
Aortic valve disease, 9
Aortic valve movements, studied by
        echocardiography, 66
Apex beat, in palpation of the
        heart, 28
Arterial hypertension, 8
Arterial pressure pulse, 49
Arterial pulsation, 26
    exaggerated, 19
    in suprasternal notch, in palpa-
        tion of the heart, 30
Arterial pulse, in mitral stenosis,
        211
Arteriovenous aneurysm of lung,
        44
Aschoff node, 201
Ascites, 9, 11
Atheromatous aorta, high, 20

Atrial ectopic beats, 102
Atrial fibrillation, 12, 102
    clinical features, 112
    in mitral stenosis, 214
    mechanism and cardiogram,
        111
    treatment, 113
    with tricuspid reflux in jugular
        venous pulse, 27
Atrial flutter, 102
    mechanism and cardiogram,
        108
    treatment, 110
    treatment with DC shock, 118
Atrial pressure pulse, 49
Atrial septal defect, 187
    atrial flutter following closure
        of, 110
Atrioventricular block, 123
    cardiogram, 126
    clinical features, 125
    definition, 123
    pathology, 124
    prognosis, 126
    radiology, 126
    treatment, 127
    types, 123
Atrio-ventricular node, 70, 73
    effect of interruption of conduc-
        tion at various levels,
        121
Atropine, 292
Augmented unipolar limb leads,
        79
Auscultation, 31
Austin Flint murmur, 44
Average heart rate, 99

Bacterial endocarditis,
    aetiology and pathology, 239
    clinical features, 240
    complications, 242
    diagnosis, 242
    prophylaxis, 243
    prognosis, 242
    treatment, 243
Ball thrombus of left atrium, as
        cause of syncope, 17
Bendrofluazide, 292

in treatment of high blood pressure, 138
Benign idiopathic pericarditis, 249
Beta-receptor blocking drugs, 293
in treatment of high blood pressure, 139
in treatment of paroxysmal atrial tachycardia, 106
Bethanidine, 294
in treatment of high blood pressure, 139, 140
Bi-ventricular hypertrophy, 12
Bigeminy, 100
Blood pressure, 47
gradients, 49
pressure, flow and resistance relationships, 48
pulse contours, 49
Blood pressure, high,
aetiological factors and mechanism, 130
biochemical investigation, 135
causes and types, 129
clinical features, 133
definition, 129
pathology, 132
prognosis, 136
treatment, 137
Breast arteries in pregnancy, enlarged, 44
Breathlessness, see Dyspnoea
Bretylium, 294
Bronchial arteries in pulmonary atresia, enlarged, 44
Bronchial asthma,
differentiation from cardiac disease, 16
differentiation from pulmonary oedema, 11
Bronchitis, winter, in mitral stenosis, 211
Bumetanide, 294
Bundle branch block, 93, 122
S-T segment abnormalities, 96

Calcification,
in the aortic knob, 59
in the ascending aorta, 59

of mitral and aortic valves, in radioscopy, 60
Cannon waves,
in atrioventricular block, 125
in jugular venous pulse, 28
in ventricular tachycardia, 116
Cardiac index, 6
Cardiac infarction,
causing ventricular fibrillation, 116
causing ventricular tachycardia, 115
involving papillary muscles, 223
Cardiac output, 6, 46
basic determinants, 2
during exercise, 3
Cardiac pulsation,
large amplitude, 5
radioscopy 60
Cardiac vectors, 82
Cardiogram waves, 77
Cardiographic abnormalities, in rheumatic fever, 204
Cardiographic deflections, significance of, 80
Cardiographic patterns after exercise, normal and abnormal, 97
Cardiomyopathies,
definition,
classification, 278
presentation, 279
metabolic and hypertrophic, 8
Cardiomyopathy, 2.
hypertrophic,
cardiac catheterization, 281
cardiogram, 280
clinical features, 280
differential diagnosis, 281
haemodynamics, 279
pathology, 279
prognosis, 281
radiology, 280
treatment, 281
restrictive,
clinical features, 282
haemodynamics, 282
pathology, 282

treatment, 282
with congestive failure,
    cardiogram, 283
    clinical features, 282
    pathology, 282
    treatment, 283
Carditis, in rheumatic fever, 203
Carotid artery, kinked, 31
Catecholamines, 2
Central cyanosis, 22
Chest leads, 80
Chest pain, as symptom, 16
Chlorthalidone,
    in treatment of congestive heart
        failure, 13
    in treatment of high blood pres-
        sure, 138
Cholesterol, serum, raised, and high
    blood pressure, 136
Chordae tendinae,
    congenital and familial abnor-
        malities of, 225
    rupture of, 224
Chorea, in rheumatic fever, 205
Cigarette smoking, and high blood
    pressure, 136
Claudication, 18
Clonidine, 294
    in treatment of high blood pres-
        sure, 139, 140
Clubbing of fingers, 19, 20
Coarctation of the aorta, 20, 31
Coarse fibrillation, 112
Coeur en sabot, 56
Congenital heart disease, 177
    parasternal systolic murmurs
        without cyanosis, differ-
        ential diagnosis, 192,
        194
    atrial septal defect, 192
    aortic stenosis, 193
    physiological murmurs of
        childhood, 192
    pulmonary stenosis, 193
    ventricular septal defect, 193
    treatment, 179
    with left-to-right shunt and com-
        bined ventricular hyper-
        trophy, 189

ventricular septal defect,
    189
    cardiogram, 191
    clinical features, 190
    haemodynamics, 189
    morbid anatomy, 189
    prognosis, 191
    radioscopy, 191
    treatment, 191
with left-to-right shunt and left
    ventricular hypertrophy,
    185
    patent ductus arteriosus, 185
    cardiogram, 186
    clinical features, 186
    haemodynamics, 185
    morbid anatomy, 185
    radiology, 186
    treatment, 186
with left-to-right shunt and right
    ventricular hypertrophy,
    187
    atrial septal defect, 187
    cardiogram, 188
    clinical features of ostium
        primum type, 189
    clinical features of ostium
        secundum type, 187
    haemodynamics, 187
    morbid anatomy, 187
    radiology, 188
    treatment 188
with left ventricular hypertrophy
    and no shunt, 179
    coarctation of the aorta, 179
    associated defects, 180
    cardiogram, 180
    clinical features, 180
    complications, 181
    haemodynamics, 179
    morbid anatomy, 179
    treatment, 181
    congenital aortic stenosis,
        181
    cardiogram, 181
    clinical features, 181
    haemodynamics, 181
    morbid anatomy, 181
    prognosis, 181

radiology, 181
treatment, 182
fibroelastosis, 182
clinical features, 182
definititon, 182
treatment, 182
with right-to-left shunt, right ventricular hypertrophy and low pulmonary flow and pressure, 196
Tetralogy of Fallot, 196
cardiogram, 199
clinical features, 198
differential diagnosis, 199
haemodynamics, 197
morbid anatomy, 196
radiology, 199
treatment, 199
with right-to-left shunt, low pulmonary blood flow and high pulmonary vascular resistance, 193
Eisenmenger's Complex 193
Eisenmenger syndrome, 193
cardiogram, 196
clinical features, 195
differential diagnosis, 196
haemodyamics, 195
radiology 196
with right ventricular hypertrophy and no shunt, 183
congenital pulmonary stenosis, 183
cardiogram, 184
clinical features, 183
haemodynamics, 183
morbid anatomy, 183
radiology, 184
treatment, 184
Congestive heart failure, 6, 11
clinical features, 12
in mitral stenosis, 214
treatment, 12
use of diuretics, 13
Conn's syndrome, 135
Continuous murmurs, 44
Convulsions, accompanying syncope, 17
Cor pulmonale, chronic, 269
cardiogram, 271
clinical features, 270
definition, 269
diagnosis, 272
haemodynamics, 269
pathology, 269
prognosis, 272
prophylaxis, 272
treatment, 273
Coronary angiography, 61
Coronary artery, abnormal connecting with right heart, 44
Coronary artery atheroma, 8
Coronary thrombosis, causing ventricular fibrillation, 116
Corrigan's sign, 231
Cyanosis, 19, 22
in congenital heart disease, 177
Cyanotic congenital heart disease, as cause of syncope, 17
studied by angiography, 60

DC Shock, failure and complications, 118
in treatment of, atrial fibrillation, 112, 113
atrial flutter, 110
paroxysmal atrial tachycardia, 105
paroxysmal atrial tachycardia with 2:1 A-V block, 107
ventricular fibrillation, 117
ventricular tachycardia, 116
nomenclature, 119
technique, 117
theory, 117
Delayed diastolic murmurs, 43
Dependent oedema, 11
Depolarisation of cells, 70
Diastolic murmurs, 41
Diastolic pressure, increased 5
Diazepam, in treatment of high blood pressure, 137
Diazoxide, 11

in treatment of high blood pressure, 140
Dicrotic wave, 50
Diffuse fibrosis, 8
Digitalis, 295
in treatment of atrial fibrillation, 113
in treatment of paroxysmal atrial tachycardia with 2:1 A-V block, 107
overdose, causing ventricular tachycardia, 115
S-T segment abnormalities, caused by, 96
Digoxin,
dose schedules, 296
effect on myocardial contractility, 2
in treatment of,
atrial flutter, 110, 111
congestive heart failure, 12
paroxysmal atrial tachycardia, 105
not to be combined with DC shock, 119
overdose, in ventricular fibrillation, 117
Direct current shock see DC shock
Disopyramide, 297
in treatment of, 110
atrial flutter, 110, 111
sinus standstill, 121
Dissecting aneurysm of the aorta,
cardiogram, 276
clinical features, 274
pathology, 274
prognosis, 276
radiology, 276
treatment, 276
Diuretics, in treatment of,
congestive heart failure, 13
high blood pressure, 138
Drugs,
action of, 290
in treatment of high blood pressure, 137
Dynamic exercise, 4
Dyspnoea, 15
in mitral stenosis, 210

paroxysmal nocturnal, 11
Dysrhythmias, 17, 100

Early diastolic murmurs, 42
Echocardiography, 63
Ectopic foci, 101
Effort dyspnoea, progressive, 10
Eisenmenger's syndrome, 272
Ejection click, 37
Electrocardiographic deflections, 77
Electrocardiography, 70
Erythema marginatum,
in rheumatic fever, 206
Exaggerated 'a' waves in jugular venous pulse, 27
Exaggerated 'y' trough in jugular venous pulse, 28
Extrasystole beat, 102

Fallot's tetralogy, 51, 56
Flow, 46
Fick formula, 50
Fick principle, 46
First heart sound, 32
in atrio-ventricular block, variation in intensity, 34
Fourth heart sound, 36
Frederickson classification of hyperlipidaemia, 147
Frusemide, 11, 297
in congestive heart failure 13, 14
Fusiform aneurysm of aorta, 59

Gallop rhythm, 10, 12, 37
General appearance of patient, 19
Glucose intolerance, and high blood pressure, 136
Glyceryl trinitrate, 297
Graham Steell murmur, 43
Guanethidine, in treatment of high blood pressure, 139, 140

Habits of patient, 17
Haemochromatosis, 8
Haemodynamics, 46
techniques, 51

Haemoptysis,   17
  in mitral stenosis,   210
Hands, warmth or coolness of,   20
Heart block, second degree,   100
Heart failure,   6
  in rheumatic fever,   205
  symptoms and signs,   15
Heart muscle, structure and pro-
        perties,   1
Heart rate,   99
Heart rhythm,   100
Heart sounds,   32
Heart valve diseases,   209
Heparin,   298
  in treatment of
        atrial fibrillation,   113
        pulmonary infarction,   263
Heredity, in high blood pres-
        sure,   132
His bundle electrocardiogram,   76
His-Purkinje cells,   73, 75
Humoral mechanism, in high
        blood pressure,   130
Hyperdynamic impulse, in palpi-
        tation of the heart,   30
Hyperdynamic ventricle,   6
Hyperkinetic   circulatory
        states,   236
  clinical features,   236
Hyperkinetic impulse,
  in palpitation of the heart,   30
Hyperkinetic ventricle,   5
Hyperlipidaemia, in ischaemic
        heart disease,   146
  treatment of,   147
Hypertension,   7, 9,
        see also Blood pressure,
        high
Hyperthyroidism,
  clinical features,   237
  treatment,   238
Hypertrophic   cardiomyopathy,
        studied by echocardiogra-
        phy,   66
Hypertrophy,   5, 9,
Hyperventilation, neurotic,   19

Immediate diastolic murmurs,   42
Infarction, see also Myocardial

infarction   8
Infra-mammary pain, left,   16
Infundibular stenosis, studied by
        angiography,   61
Intracardiac myxoma, as cause of
        syncope,   17
Intracranial lesions, causing T wave
        abnormalities,   98
Intravenous pyelography,   136
Intraventricular block,   122
Ischaemic cardiac pain,   16
Ischaemic fibrosis or infarction
        confined to papillary mus-
        cles,   223
Ischaemic heart disease,   8
  aetiology,   145
  chronic   ischaemic   heart
        disease,   174
  clinical presentation,   150
  definition,   146
  haemodynamics,   149
  morbid anatomy,   148
  myocardial infarction,   157
Ischaemic kidney, in high blood
        pressure,   131
Isoprenaline,   298
  effect on myocardial contractil-
        ity,   2, 3

Jugular venous pressure,   10
  assessment of,   23
  in mitral stenosis,   212
Junctional ectopic beats,   107
Junctional rhythm,   100, 107
Junctional tachycardia,
  clinical features,   108
  mechanism   and   cardio-
        gram,   107
  treatment,   108

Kidney, ischaemic, in high blood
        pressure,   132
Kinidin durules, see Quinidine

Left anterior hemi-block,   122
Left atrial enlargement,   56
Left atrial hypertrophy,   87
Left atrial pressure,
  high,   11

normal, 9
Left atrial thrombus or myxoma, studied by echocardiography, 68
Left axis deviation, 84
Left bundle branch block, 93
Left heart catheterization,
by retrograde arterial route, 52
by trans-septal route, 52
Left heart failure, 6, 8
Left infra-mammary pain, 16
Left posterior hemi-block, 122
Left ventricular angiography and aortography, 61
Left ventricular end-diastolic pressure, 9
Left ventricular enlargement, 57
Left ventricular function, studied by echocardiography, 68
Left ventricular hypertrophy, 10
abnormalities of QRS complex, 90
in palpitation of the heart, 29
S-T segment abnormalities, 96
voltage in, 91
with high blood pressure, 136
Lignocaine, 299
in treatment of ventricular ectopic beats, 115
in treatment of ventricular tachycardia, 116
Liver enlargement, 7, 11
gross, 9
Lone atrial fibrillation, 112, 113
Low potassium, effect on electrocardiogram, 98
Low voltage of the cardiogram, 93, 94

Maladie de Roger, 190
Mean QRS vector, 82
direction of, 84
Mean T wave vector, 86
Medical history of patient, 17
Methyl Dopa, in treatment of high blood pressure, 138,140
Mexiletine, 299
Mid-diastolic murmurs, 43

Mid-systolic murmurs, 38
Migratory arthritis in rheumatic fever, 203
Mitral reflux, 7, 9, 215
cardiogram, 218
complications, 218
clinical features, 217
echocardiography, 66
haemodynamics, 216
pathology, 215
prognosis, 218
radiology, 218
treatment, 218
Mitral reflux, non-rheumatic, and papillary muscle dysfunction, 220
aetiology and pathology, 221
clinical features, 223
differential diagnosis, 225
haemodynamics, 222
normal function of papillary muscles and chordae, 221
prognosis and treatment, 226
Mitral stenosis, 9, 16, 17, 209
cardiac catheterization, 213
cardiogram, 212
complications, 214
differential diagnosis, 214
echocardiography, 65
haemodynamics, 209
morbid anatomy, 209
prognosis, 215
radiology, 213
treatment, 215
with atrial fibrillation, 113
with reflux
angiocardiography, 227
clinical features, 226
haemodynamics, 226
pathology, 226
prognosis, 227
radiology, 227
treatment, 227
Mitral valve disease, 10
Mitral valve function, assessed by angiography, 61
Mitral valve movements, studied by echocardiography 64

Mitral valve obstruction, by ball thrombus or myxoma, 9
Mitral valvitis, in rheumatic fever, 203
Mobitz type I and II blocks, 123, 126
Morphine, 11
Myocardial cell, action potential, 75
Myocardial contractility, 2
Myocardial disease, 8
Myocardial function, direct impairment, 8
Myocardial infarction, in ischaemic heart disease, 149, 157
  cardiac infarction without abnormal Q waves, 161
  cardiogenic shock, 173
  cardiogram, 159
  clinical features, 158
  complications, 167
  differential diagnosis, 165
  haemodynamics, 157
  left bundle branch block, 163
  pathology, 157
  rehabilitation, 173
  reliability of cardiogram, 164
  right bundle branch block, 162
  serum enzymes in myocardial infarction, 164
  treatment, 169
  treatment of complications, 171
Myofibrils, 1
Myopathies, hereditary neurological, 8
Myosin filaments, 1
Myxoedema, 8
Myxoma of the atria,
  clinical features, 253
  differential diagnosis, 254
  echocardiography, 254
  pathology, 253
  radiology, 254

Neurogenic mechanism, in high blood pressure, 130
Nodal ectopic beats, see Junctional ectopic beats

Nodal rhythm, see Junctional rhythm
Noradrenaline, effect on myocardial contractility, 2, 3

Obesity, and high blood pressure, 136
Obstructive cardiomyopathy, deformities due to, studied by angiography, 61
Oedema, 17
Orthopnoea, 11
Osler's nodes, 241
Oxprenolol, 300
  in treatment of high blood pressure, 139
Oxygen, 300

P wave, 78
  abnormalities, 86
  genesis, 87
  in atrial ectopic beats, 102
P-R interval abnormalities, 88
Pacemaker,
  in atrioventricular block, 127
  in sinus standstill, 121
Palpitations, 16, 28
Pan-systolic murmurs, 40
Paroxysmal atrial tachycardia,
  mechanism and cardiogram, 103
  treatment, 104
  with 2:1 A-V block,
    clinical features, 106
    mechanism and cardiogram, 106
    treatment, 107
Paroxysmal tachycardia, 89
  reciprocating, 102
Patent ductus arteriosus, 44
Pathological stress, 4
Penicillin in treatment of rheumatic fever, 207
Percussion, 31
Percussion wave, 49
Percutaneous left ventricular puncture, 51
Perhexiline, 301
Pericardial constriction, 9

cardiogram, 251
clinical features, 250
differential diagnosis, 251
haemodynamics, 250
pathology, 250
prognosis, 251
radiology, 251
treatment, 252
Pericardial effusion, 9, 59
angiography, 61
echocardiography, 67
Pericarditis,
aetiology, 245
cardiogram, 245
clinical features, 245
differential diagnosis, 248
echocardiogram, 247
in rheumatic fever, 204
paracentesis, 247
pathology, 245
radiology, 246
S-T segment abnormalities, 96
treatment, 248
types of, distinguishing features, 248
Peripheral cyanosis, 22
Peripheral vasodilators, in treatment of high blood pressure, 139
Phaeochromocytoma, 142
clinical features, 142
diagnosis, 142
differential diagnosis, 143
treatment, 143
Phenoxy-benzamine *see* phentolamine
Phentolamine, 3, 4
in treatment of phaeochromocytoma, 143
Phenytoin, 301
Phlebography, 259
Pleural effusions, 9, 11
Polarisation of cells, 70
Polycythaemia, 19
Potassium, 301
depletion,
causing S-T wave abnormalities 98
from use of digitalis, 295

in polarisation of cells, 70
in ventricular fibrillation, 117
Practolol, in treatment of,
atrial flutter, 110
paroxysmal tachycardia, 106
ventricular tachycardia, 116
Prazosin, in treatment of high blood pressure, 139
Pre-excitation syndrome, 88, 102
Pregnancy and rheumatic heart disease, 218
pulmonary oedema, 219
contraception and sterilization, 220
Pregnancy and the heart,
haemodynamics and clinical features, 236
Prenylamine, 302
Procainamide, 302
Propranolol, 303
effect on cardiac output, 3, 4
in treatment of,
atrial flutter, 110
high blood pressure, 139, 140
phaeochromocytoma, 143
sinus standstill, 121
ventricular tachycardia, 116
Psychogenic origin, symptoms of, 19
Pulmonary angiography, 257
Pulmonary arterial hypertension due to increased flow,
hyperkinetic, 265
clinical features, 266
radiology, 266
vaso-occlusive, 266
cardiogram, 267
clinical features, 266
differential diagnosis, 267
patho-physiology, 266
radiology, 267
Pulmonary artery,
enlargement of, 58
in palpitation of the heart, 30
Pulmonary embolism,
clinical features, 256
haemodynamics, 255
pathology, 255

Pulmonary hypertension, 5, 7, 264
Pulmonary infarction,
  clinical features, 262
  differential diagnosis, 262
  prognosis, 263
  prophylaxis, 263
  radiology, 262
  treatment, 263
Pulmonary oedema, 7, 9
  cardiogram, 10
  diagnosis, 10
  radiology, 10
  treatment, 11
  use of morphine, 11
Pulmonary valve stenosis, angiography, 61
Pulmonary venous hypertension with passive pulmonary arterial hypertension,
  clinical features, 265
  haemodynamics, 264
  pathology, 264
  radiology, 265
Pulse,
  amplitude of, 20
  jugular venous, 25, 27
  normal arterial, diagram of, 21
  quick rising, 20
  radial or brachial, 20
  slow rising, 21
  wave form of, 20
Pulsus paradoxus, 246

QRS axis, normal range of, 85
QRS complex, 78
  abnormalities, 90
QRS in atrial ectopic beats, 102
QRS vectors, 82
  at 0.04 seconds, 84
Quinidine, 303
  in cardiography, 97
  in treatment of atrial flutter, 111

Radioactive fibrinogen, use of, 259
Radiology, 54
  accuracy of, 60

Radioscopy, 60
Raised serum cholesterol and high blood pressure, 136
Raynaud's phenomenon, 22
Reciprocating rhythms, 101
Re-entry, diagram of, 101
Relative refractory period, 101
Renin, in high blood pressure, 130
Repolarisation of cells, 70, 71
Reserpine in treatment of high blood pressure, 140
Resistance, 47
Resting potential
Resuscitation, 284
  aftercare, 286
  indications, 284
  method, 284
Rheumatic fever, 201
  aetiology, 201
  clinical features, 203
  definition, 201
  differential diagnosis, 206
  pathology, 201
  prognosis, 207
  prophylaxis, 207
  treatment, 207
Rheumatic heart disease, murmurs, 12
Rheumatic pericarditis, 248
Rhonchi, 16
Right atrial enlargement, 55
Right atrial hypertrophy, 86
Right atrial tumours, diagnosed by angiography, 61
Right axis deviation, 84
Right bundle branch block, 93
  with left anterior hemi-block, 123
  with left posterior hemi-block, 123
Right heart catheterization, 51
Right heart failure, 6, 7
Right ventricular enlargement, 56
Right ventricular hypertrophy, 92
  in palpitation of the heart, 30
Rogitine, in treatment of phaeochromocytoma, 143

ST segment, 78

S-T segment waves, abnormalities, 94
Salt intake, restriction of, 13
Sarcomeres, 1
Second heart sound, 35
Seldinger technique, 51
Serum cholesterol, raised and high blood pressure, 136
Shunts, 50
    in congenital heart disease, 177
'Sick Sinus Syndrome', 120
Sino-atrial block, 120
Sino-atrial node, 70, 73
Sinus arrhythmia, 100
    of valsalva, 44
        ruptured, 44
    standstill, 120
        clinical features, 121
        mechanism and cardiogram, 120
        treatment, 121
Sodium, in polarisation of cells, 70
Sorbide nitrate, 32
Spironolactone, 304
Sputum, pink, frothy, 10
Standard leads, 78
Starling's law of the heart, 2
Static work for patients with heart disease, 4
Stenosis, pulmonary or aortic, 17
Stethoscope, choice of, 31
Stoke Adams attack, 127
Streptokinase, 305
    in pulmonary infarction, 263
Subclavian-pulmonary anastomosis, 44
Sub-cutaneous nodules in rheumatic fever, 206
Suprasternal puncture of the aorta, pulmonary artery and left atrium, 51
Supraventricular tachycardia, 100, 105
Sympathetic activity, 2
Symptoms and signs, 15
    of psychogenic origin, 19
Syncope, 17
Systemic emboli, in mitral stenosis, 211
Systemic hypertension, 5
Systemic venous pressure, 7
Systolic clicks, 37
Systolic murmurs, 39

T wave, 78
    abnormalities, 97
    vectors, 82
Ta wave, 75, 78
Tachycardia, 2, 10, 99
Third heart sound, 35
Thrombo-embolism of vascular bed, 266
Thyroid disease, 22
Thyrotoxicosis, 23
Tidal wave, 50
Transient heart block, 17
Transmembrane action potentials, 71, 73
Tricuspid reflux, 8
    aetiology, 232
    clinical features, 233
    haemodynamics, 232
    pathology, 232
    prognosis, 233
    radiology, 233
    treatment, 233
Tricuspid stenosis,
    aetiology, 234
    cardiogram, 235
    clinical features, 234
    differential diagnosis, 235
    haemodynamics, 234
    pathology, 234
    prognosis and treatment, 235
    radiology, 234
Trinitrate, response to, 16
Triple rhythm, 37
Tuberculous pericarditis, 248

U wave, 78
Ultra-sound, use of, 260
Unipolar limb leads, 79
Unipolar versus vector theory, 80
Urokinase, 305

V leads, 80
    galvanometer connection of, 81

Vagal activity, 2
Valsalva manoeuvre, 6, 104
Vascular bed,
    obliterated by chest disease,
        266
    thrombo-embolism of, 266
Vaso-constriction in pulmonary
        arterial hypertension,
        266
Vaso-vagal faint, 17
Venous hum, 44
Venous pressure,
    atrial and pulmonary, 7
    pulmonary and systemic, 9
Venous pulsation, 20, 24
Ventimask, 300
    in chronic cor pulmonale, 273
Ventricle,
    dilatation of, 5
    failing, 7
    hyperdynamic, 6
    hyperkinetic, 5
Ventricular aneurysms, S-T seg-
        ment abnormalities, 96
Ventricular ectopic (premature)
        beats,
    mechanism and cardiogram,
        114
    multifocal, 100

    treatment, 115
Ventricular fibrillation,
    clinical features, 116
    mechanism and cardiogram,
        116
    treatment, 117
        with DC shock, 118
Ventricular hypertrophy, 90
Ventricular tachycardia, 100
    clinical features, 115
    mechanism and cardiogram,
        115
    treatment, 116
Verapamil, 305
    in reciprocating tachycardia,
        106

Warfarin sodium, 306
    in treatment of atrial fibrilla-
        tion, 113
Water-hammer pulse, 20
    in atrio ventricular block, 125
    with Austin Flint murmur, 44
Wenckebach's phenomenon, 88,
        123
Wheeziness, 16
Wolff-Parkinson-White syndrome,
        88, 102